Basic Electrocardiography

NORMAL AND ABNORMAL ECG PATTERNS

A. Bayés de Luna, MD, FESC, FACC

Professor of Medicine, Universidad Autonoma Barcelona
Director of Institut Catala de Cardiologia
Hospital Santa Creu I Sant Pau
St. Antoni M. Claret 167
Director Cardiac Department – H. Quiron. Barcelona
ES-08025
Barcelona
Spain

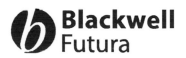
Blackwell
Futura

© 2007 A. Bayés de Luna
Published by Blackwell Publishing
Blackwell Futura is an imprint of Blackwell Publishing

Blackwell Publishing, Inc., 350 Main Street, Malden, Massachusetts 02148-5020, USA
Blackwell Publishing Ltd, 9600 Garsington Road, Oxford OX4 2DQ, UK
Blackwell Science Asia Pty Ltd, 550 Swanston Street, Carlton, Victoria 3053, Australia

First published 2007

1   2007

ISBN: 978-1-4051-7570-8

Library of Congress Cataloging-in-Publication Data

Bayes de Luna, Antonio.
    Basic electrocardiography : normal and abnormal ECG patterns / Antoni Bayes de Luna.
        p. ; cm.
    Includes bibliographical references and index.
    ISBN 978-1-4051-7570-8
    1. Electrocardiography.   2. Heart – Diseases – Diagnosis.   I. Title.
    [DNLM: 1. Electrocardiography.   2. Electrocardiography – methods.
    WG 140 B357b 2007]
    RC683.5.E5B324 2007
    616.1′207547 – dc22

                                    2007006646

A catalogue record for this title is available from the British Library

Commissioning Editor: Gina Almond
Development Editor: Fiona Pattison
Editorial Assistant: Victoria Pitman

Set in 9.5/12pt Palatino by Aptara Inc., New Delhi, India
Printed and bound in Singapore by Fabulous Printers Pte Ltd.

For further information on Blackwell Publishing, visit our website:
www.blackwellcardiology.com

Basic
Electrocardiography

NORMAL AND ABNORMAL
ECG PATTERNS

Contents

Foreword

Basic Electrocardiography: Normal and Abnormal ECG Patterns is not an additional regular textbook on electrocardiography. Professor Antoni Bayés de Luna, the author of the present textbook is a world-wide renowned electrocardiographer and clinical cardiologist who has contributed to our knowledge and understanding of electrocardiology over the years. In the present textbook, he shares with us his vast experience and knowledge, summarising the traditional concepts of electrocardiography and vectrocardiography combined with current updates on the most recent developments correlating electrocardiographic patterns with magnetic resonance imaging. This textbook is of particular value to the American physicians and healthcare providers, as it exposes the reader to the Mexican, Argentinean and European schools of electrocardiography, which some of the earlier textbooks have tended to overlook.

The present textbook provides a concise summary of the classical and modern concepts of electrocardiology and provides 22 cases covering a wide spectrum of normal variations and abnormal electrocardiographic findings. In these cases Dr. Bayés de Luna explains his approach for interpreting the electrocardiogram and integrating it with the clinical findings.

In conclusion, this textbook is an asset for every cardiologist, internist, primary care physician, as well as medical students and other healthcare providers interested in broadening their skills in electrocardiography.

Yochai Birnbaum, MD
Edward D. and Sally M. Futch Professor of Medicine
Biochemistry and Molecular Biology
Medical Director, Cardiac Intensive Care Unit
Medical Director, the Heart Station
The Division of Cardiology
The University of Texas Medical Branch

CHAPTER 1

Introduction

The electrocardiogram (ECG), introduced into clinical practice more than 100 years ago by Einthoven, constitutes a lineal recording of the heart's electrical activity that occurs successively over time. An atrial depolarisation wave (P wave), a ventricular depolarisation wave (QRS complex) and a ventricular repolarisation wave (T wave) are successively recorded for each cardiac cycle (Figures 1A–C). As these different waves are recorded from different sites (leads) the morphology varies (Figure 2). Nevertheless, the sequence is always P–QRS–T. An ECG curve recorded from an electrode facing the left ventricle is shown in Figure 1D. Depending on the heart rate, the interval between waves of one cycle and another is variable.

Other different forms of recording cardiac activity (vectorcardiography, body mapping, etc.) exist [1]. Vectorcardiography (VCG) represents electrical activity by different loops originating from the union of the heads of multiple vectors of atrial depolarisation (P loop), ventricular depolarisation (QRS loop), and ventricular repolarisation (T loop). A close correlation exists between VCG loops and the ECG curve. Therefore, one may deduct ECG morphology on the basis of the morphology of VCG loop and vice versa. This is due to loop–hemifield correlation theory (see p. 10). According to this correlation (Figures 16, 18 and 21), the morphology of different waves (P, QRS and T) recorded from different sides (leads) varies (Figure 2). As the heart is a three-dimensional organ, projection of the loops with their maximum vectors in two planes, frontal and horizontal, on the positive and the negative hemifield* of each lead is required to ascertain exactly the loop's location and allow deducting ECG morphology (Figures 3 and 4). The morphology of ECG depends not only on the maximum vector of a given loop but also on its rotation (Figure 4). This represents the importance of considering the loop and not only its maximum vector to explain the ECG morphology.

---

*The positive and the negative hemifield of each lead are obtained by drawing lines perpendicular to each lead, passing through the centre of the heart. The positive hemifield is located in the area of positive part of the lead, and the negative hemifield in the negative part. In Figure 4 the positive hemifield is the area located between −90° and +90° passing through 0°, and the positive hemifield of lead VF is the area located between 0° and 180° passing through +90°. The other part of the electrical field corresponds to the negative hemifield of each lead (see p. 10).

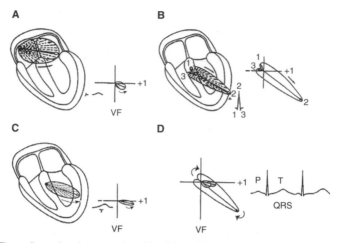

Figure 1 Three-dimensional perspective of the P loop (A), QRS loop with its three representative vectors (B) and T loop (C), and their projection on the frontal plane with the correlation loop–ECG morphology. (D) Global correlation between the P, QRS and T loops and ECG morphology on the frontal plane recorded in a lead facing the left ventricle free wall (lead I).

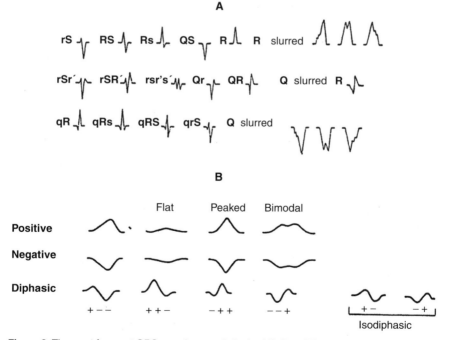

Figure 2 The most frequent QRS complex morphologies (A), P and T waves morphologies (B).

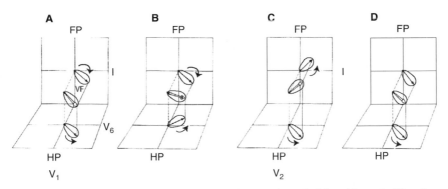

Figure 3 A loop with its maximum vector directed downwards, to the left and forwards (A) and another with its maximum vector directed downwards, to the left and backwards (B) have the same projections on the frontal plane (FP) but different projections on the horizontal plane (HP). On the other hand, a loop with the maximum vector directed upwards, to the left and forwards (C) and another with the maximum vector directed downwards, to the left and forwards (D) produce the same projection on the HP, but different projections on the FP.

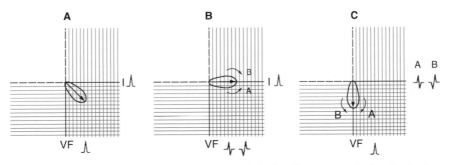

Figure 4 If the maximum vector of a loop falls in the limit of positive and negative hemifields of a certain lead, an isodiphasic deflection is recorded. However, according to the direction of loop rotation the QRS complex may be positive–negative or negative–positive (see examples for leads VF and I in the case of maximum vector directed to 0° (B) and +90° (C)). The loop with maximum vector at 45° (A) always fails in the positive hemifield of I and VF, independently of the sense of rotation.

VCG is rarely used in current clinical practice; however, it is highly useful in understanding ECG morphologies and in teaching electrocardiography. Later in this book we will explain in more detail how the loops originate and how their projection in frontal and horizontal planes explains the ECG morphologies in different leads.

CHAPTER 2

Usefulness and limitations of electrocardiography

ECG is the technique of choice in the study of patients with chest pain, syncope, palpitations and acute dyspnoea, and is crucial for the diagnosis of cardiac arrhythmias, conduction disturbances, pre-excitation syndromes and channelopathies. It is also very important for assessing the evolution and response to treatment of all types of heart diseases and other diseases, and different situations such as electrolytic disorders, drug administration, athletes, surgical evaluation, etc. Additionally, it is useful for epidemiologic studies and screening (check-up).

Despite its invaluable usefulness if used correctly, electrocardiography may induce mistakes if one excessively trusts on an ECG recording of normal appearance. Sometimes, bowing to the 'magical' power of ECG, physicians caring for a patient with chest pain of doubtful origin may state: 'Let's have an ECG recording done so that we may solve the problem'. It must be remembered that a high percentage of patients with coronary heart disease, in the absence of chest pain, show a normal ECG recording and that even in acute coronary syndromes ECG is normal or borderline in approximately 5–10% of cases, and without symptoms especially in its early phase. Furthermore, ECG may be normal months or years after a myocardial infarction. From the above, it can be inferred that a normal ECG does not imply any 'life insurance' as a patient may die from cardiac causes even on the same day a normal recording is taken. However, it is evident that in the absence of clinical findings or family history of sudden death, the possibility of this occurring is, in fact, very remote.

On the other hand, on occasions some subtle ECG abnormalities with no evidence of heart disease may be observed. Clearly, in such cases one must be cautious, and before considering this to be a non-specific abnormality, ischaemic heart disease, channelopathies (long QT, Brugada's syndrome, etc.) or pre-excitation syndromes should be ruled out. Therefore, it is necessary to read the ECG recordings while bearing in mind the clinical setting and, if necessary, taking sequential recordings.

In addition, normal variants may be observed in the ECG recording, which are related to constitutional habits, chest malformations, age, etc. Even transient abnormalities may be detected owing to a number of causes (hyperventilation, hypothermia, glucose or alcohol intake, ionic abnormalities, effect of certain drugs, etc.).

Electrocardiography has become even more important than it was at the beginning. In the twenty-first century, ECG is not only a technique used to diagnose an abnormal pattern, but also serves for risk stratification in many clinical situations such as acute and chronic heart disease, cardiomyopathies, etc., and provides insights into basic electrophysiology by recognising abnormalities at a molecular level such as channelopathies [2].

These facts should be borne in mind before starting to learn a technique such as electrocardiography, so that the significant usefulness of the clinical aspects is not left aside, since ECG assessment need to be done considering the clinical setting.

In this book, we explain the origin of normal ECG and the normal and abnormal ECG patterns. The importance of surface ECG in the diagnosis of arrhythmias is not shown and will be done in another book. We recommend consulting our textbook on clinical electrocardiography [1] and our Internet course (www.cursoecg.com).

CHAPTER 3

Electrophysiological principles

The origin of ECG morphology

The origin of ECG morphology [1,3–7] may be explained by two theories: the electroionic changes generated during cardiac depolarisation and repolarisation and the sum of subendocardial and subepicardial transmembrane action potential.

Electroionic changes during depolarisation and repolarisation
Depolarisation and repolarisation of cardiac cells

There are two types of cardiac cells (Figure 5): myocardial contractile cells and specific conduction system (SCS) cells. The latter are responsible for generation (automatism capacity) and transmission (conduction capacity) of a stimulus to contractile cells. Cells with the highest automatism are those of a sinus node since they present more rapid diastolic depolarisation (see below and Figure 5). Contractile cells are polarised during the resting phase, which indicates that a balance exists between positive charges outside (due to prevalence of positive ions particularly Na^+ and Ca^{2+}) and negative charges inside (due to prevalence of negative non-diffusible anions despite the presence of positive K ions). This constant potential difference between outside and inside the cell during the resting phase constitutes the diastolic transmembrane potential (DTP) (Figure 6). Therefore, contractile cells have a rectilinear DTP; in contrast, cells of the specific conduction system have a DTP that shows spontaneous depolarisation (ascending DTP slope), which is most rapid in sinus node (Figure 5).

When a cell or different structures of the heart are stimulated, a transmembrane action potential (TAP) curve, representing the depolarisation and repolarisation processes (activation), is formed just when the DTP curve reaches the threshold. This happens spontaneously in the SCS cells and more rapidly in sinus node cells since these are cells with the highest automaticity (Figure 5). In contractile cells (atrial and ventricular muscle cells) that present rectilinear DTP, a TAP is formed only when they receive the propagated stimulus from a neighbouring cell (Figure 5).

Ionic changes accounting for TAP generation in contractile ventricular myocardium (a cell or all left ventricle, if the latter is considered to be an enormous cell responsible for the greater part of a human ECG) are shown in a Figure 7. During depolarisation (phases 0 and 1 of TAP), positive charges move from outside to inside the cell, first through the fast channel of Na^+ and later that of $Ca^{2+}Na^+$. During repolarisation of the cell or left ventricle (phases 2 and 3

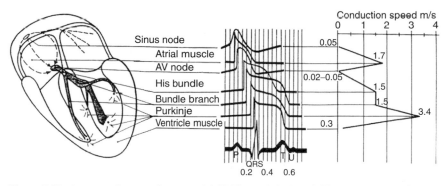

Figure 5 The transmembrane action potential (TAP) morphologies of different structures of the specialised conduction system, and atrial and ventricular muscles, the correlation with the curve of the ECG, and the impulse conduction speed through these structures.

of TAP), positive charges (K^+) exit from the cell to compensate for the extracellular negativity. After phase 3 of TAP, an electric but not ionic balance is achieved. An active mechanism (ionic pump – see Figure 7) is required to restore the ionic balance.

The dipole–vector–loop–hemifield correlation

A pair of electric charges termed **dipole** is formed in both depolarisation (−+) and repolarisation (+−) processes (TAP). This results from ionic changes that explain the formation of TAP (Figure 7). These dipoles have a **vectorial expression**, with the head of the vector located in the positive part of a dipole. An electrode that faces the head of the vector records positive deflexion regardless of whether this dipole approaches the electrode or moves away. How the cellular and ventricular electrograms are formed is shown in Figures 8 and 9. In human ECG, the repolarisation wave (T wave) is positive since physiologically there is less perfusion in the subendocardial zone and the process of

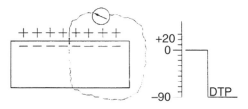

Figure 6 Two microelectrodes placed on the surface of a myocardial fibre during the resting phase record a horizontal reference line (RL) (baseline), indicating the absence of differences in potential on the cell surface. When one of the microelectrodes is inserted into the interior of the cell, there is a movement below the baseline corresponding to the difference in potential between the cell exterior (+) (Na, Ca) and interior (−) (predominance of non-diffusible anions). (A) This line, the diastolic transmembrane potential (DTP), is stable in contractile cells and with more or less upsloping in automatic cells (see Figure 5).

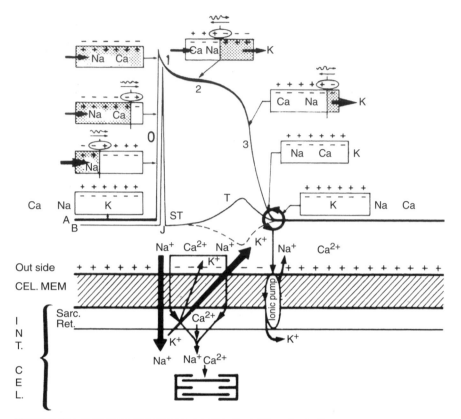

Figure 7 The electroionic correlation in a contractile cell (see the text).

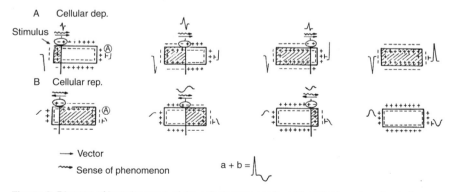

Figure 8 Diagram of how the curve of the cell electrogram (a + b) originates according to the dipole theory. (A) Cell depolarisation; (B) cell repolarisation (see the text).

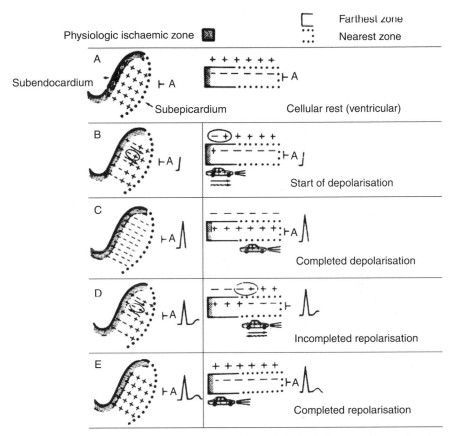

Figure 9 Depolarisation (QRS) and repolarisation (T) morphologies in the normal human heart. The figures to the left show a view of the free left ventricular wall from above, and only the distribution of the charges on the external surface of this enormous left ventricular cell is seen. Right column shows the lateral view in which the intracellular changes in the electrical charges are observed. With electrode A in the epicardium the QRS and T are positive because in both cases (depolarisation and repolarisation) electrode A faces the head of a vector although during depolarisation the direction of phenomenon goes towards the electrode (B and C) and during repolarisation moves away (D and E). Nevertheless, in both cases the lights of a car, as an example, are directed towards the electrode.

repolarisation always starts in the more perfused zone. Therefore, in human ECG, this process begins in the subepicardium, the opposite of what occurs at the cell level (Figures 8 and 9).

P, QRS and **T loops** are formed from the union of the heads of all depolarisation and repolarisation vectors indicating the way of electric stimulus during these processes (Figure 1). As already stated, only the projection on two planes, frontal and horizontal, may provide exact information as to the direction of respective electric forces (in frontal plane, upwards–downwards and right–left, and in horizontal plane, right–left and anterior–posterior) (Figure 3). Each of these loops has its **maximum vector** that is considered to be the sum of all instantaneous vectors (Figures 1 and 3) and expresses the magnitude and general direction of a loop. Nevertheless, the morphology of a loop, especially its initial and terminal part as well as loop rotation (clockwise or anti-clockwise), represents a significant additional value. Thanks to careful loop analysis, ECG morphologies may be better understood (Figures 1D, 4, 16, 18 and 21).

The sum of subendocardial and subepicardial TAP

The other approach to **understanding ECG morphology is based on the concept that the TAP of a cell or the left ventricle (considered as a huge cell that originates the human ECG) is equal to the sum of subendocardial and subepicardial TAPs.** How this occurs is shown in Figure 10 (see the caption). This concept is useful for understanding how the ECG patterns of ischaemia and injury are generated, although these morphologies may also be explained by the ischaemic and injury vector concept (see sections 'Electrocardiographic pattern of ischaemia' and 'Electrocardiographic pattern of injury' in Chapter 11).

The leads and hemifields

The ECG presents different morphologies when we record it from different sites, named leads. We currently use six frontal (I, II, III, VR, VL, VF) and six horizontal (V1__V6) leads. There are three bipolar leads I, II and III in the frontal plane, which, according to the Einthoven law, should satisfy condition II = I + III. These three leads form the Einthoven triangle (Figure 11A). Bailey, shifting the three leads towards the centre, obtained a reference figure (**Bailey's triaxial system**) (Figure 12A). There are also three monopolar leads (VR, VL and VF) in the frontal plane (Figure 11B). By adding these three leads to Bailey's triaxial system, Bailey's hexaxial system is obtained (Figure 12B). How the projection of different vectors (or loops) gives different morphologies in leads I, II and III is depicted in Figure 11C. On a horizontal plane, there are six monopolar leads (V1 to V6)* (Figure 13).

If lines perpendicular to the frontal and horizontal leads are drawn passing through the centre of the heart, **positive and negative hemifields** of these leads may be obtained (Figure 14). The lead I positive hemifield extends from +90° to −90° passing through 0°; that of lead II extends from −30° to +150° passing through +60°, that of lead III from +30° to −150° passing through +120°, that of VR extends from +120° to −60° passing through −150°, that of VL extends from −120° to +60° passing through −30°, that of VF extends from 0° to ±180° passing through +90°, that of V2 from 0° to 180° passing through +90°, and that of V6 extends from −90° to +90° passing through 0°. The rest of the hemifields corresponding to the horizontal plane leads can be obtained in

---

*On some occasions of right ventricular infarction, right precordial leads may be useful for diagnosis (Figure 74).

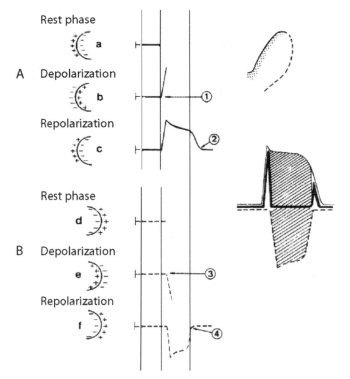

Figure 10 Correlation between TAP of the farthest subendocardium (A) and the nearest subepicardium (B) part of the left ventricle and ECG curve. 1. Beginning of the depolarisation in the farthest zone. 2. End of repolarisation in the farthest zone. 3. Beginning of depolarisation in the nearest zone. 4. End of repolarisation in the nearest zone. At the end of depolarisation (b), in the farthest zone (subendocardial TAP) (A), the electrode is confronted with this part depolarised, that is, negative on the outside and positive on the inside, and as an electrode faces the positive charges of inside an ascendent TAP phase 0 is recorded. At the end of repolarisation (c), the electrode faces internal negativity because repolarisation has concluded and the curve returns to the isoelectric line. In the case of nearest part of left ventricle (subepicardial TAP) (B) the opposite occurs. When this TAP depolarises (e), which occurs later than in the subendocardial zone, this zone presents external negativity. The electrode faces this negativity and phase 0 is inscribed as negative. When this zone has repolarised (f), as it takes place earlier than in the subendocardial zone, since in subendocardium a physiological ischaemia exists and repolarisation starts in less ischaemic zone, the electrode is confronted with positive external charges since repolarisation has concluded, and the subepicardial TAP curve returns to the isoelectric line. The first and the last parts of the sum of both TAPs produce the QRS complex and T wave. The rest of two TAPs is cancelled and seen as isoelectric line (ST segment).

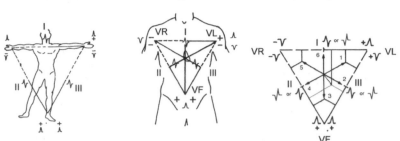

Figure 11 (A) Einthoven's triangle. (B) Einthoven's triangle superimposed on a human thorax. Observe the positive (continuous line) and negative (dotted line) part of each lead. (C) Different vectors (from 1 to 6) produce different projections according to their location. For example, vector 1 has a positive projection in lead I, diphasic in II and negative in III while vector 3 is diphasic in I, positive in II and III. For example, vector 1 has a positive deflection in I, diphasic in II and negative in III, and vector 3 is diphasic in 1 and positive in II and III. In both cases II = I + III. A vector located to +60° originates a positive deflection in I, II and III but also with II = I + III.

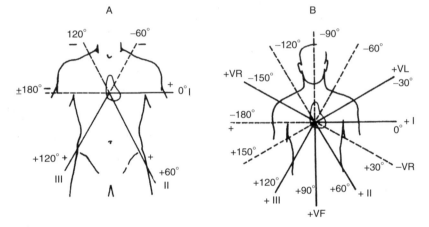

Figure 12 (A) Bailey's triaxial system. (B) Bailey's hexaxial system (see the text).

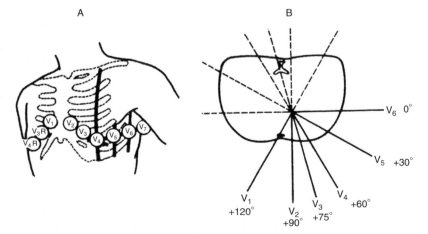

Figure 13 (A) Sites where the explorer electrodes are located in unipolar precordial leads, and (B) sites where positive poles of the six precordial leads are located.

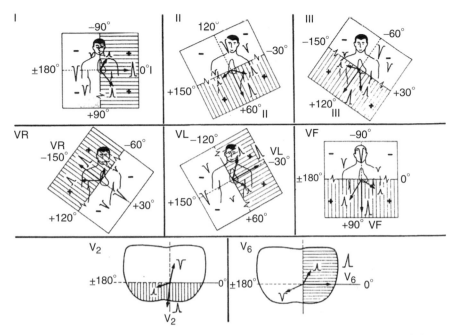

Figure 14 Positive and negative hemifields of the six frontal plane leads and the horizontal plane leads: depending on the magnitude and direction of the different vectors (which represent the corresponding loops), positive and negative deflections with different voltages are originated (see the text).

the same manner, drawing lines that are perpendicular to the corresponding lead, passing through the centre of the heart (Figure 14). In all the cases the negative hemifields are opposed to the positive ones.

A loop of P, QRS or T or its maximum vector located in the positive or the negative hemifield, or on the borderline between both hemifields in any of the 12 leads, gives rise, respectively, to a positive deflection, negative deflection, or isodiphasic deflection of P, QRS or T waves in that given lead. A isodiphasic deflection has a maximum vector but may have a different morphology; it can be positive–negative or negative–positive, according to the direction of the loop rotation that represents the path that the stimulus follows (Figure 4). The degree of positivity or negativity depends on two factors: the magnitude and the direction of the loop or vector. With the same magnitude, the vectorial force that is directed towards the positive or the negative pole in a certain lead originates positivity or negativity, respectively; with the same direction, the loop or vector with a greater magnitude will cause a greater positivity or negativity.

> The projection of P, QRS and T loops on positive and negative hemifields of different leads in frontal and horizontal planes explains the morphology of ECG, and according to the rotation of a loop the morphology may be ± or −/+ (Figures 4, 16, 18 and 21).

Activation sequence of the heart and ECG

The electrocardiographic tracing corresponds to the activation sequence (depolarisation + repolarisation) of the heart starting with the stimulus that arises in the sinus node since this is the structure with greater automaticity up to the ventricular Purkinje net through the specific conduction system (Figure 5). The

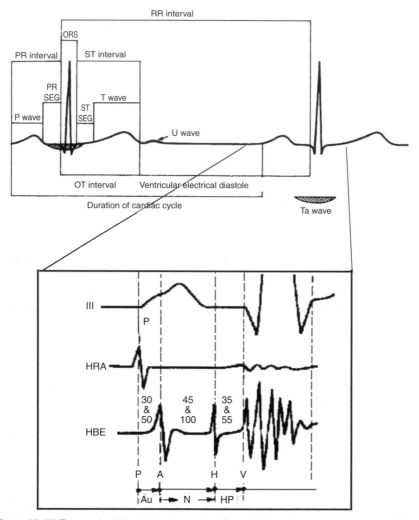

Figure 15 (A) Temporal relationship between the different ECG waves and nomenclature of the various intervals and segments. Ta wave: T wave of atrial repolarisation (see the text). (B) Observe the different spaces of the PR interval. HRA: high right atrium. HBE: His bundle electrogram. PA interval: from the upper right atrium – onset of the P wave in the surface ECG – to the first rapid lower right atrial deflection; this represents right intra-atrial conduction (Au) and its normal value oscillates between 30 and 50 ms. AH interval: from the first rapid deflection of the lower atrial electrocardiogram (A) until the bundle of His (H) deflection; this represents intranodal conduction (N) and its normal value oscillates between 45 and 100 ms. The value of HV interval ranges between 35 and 55 ms.

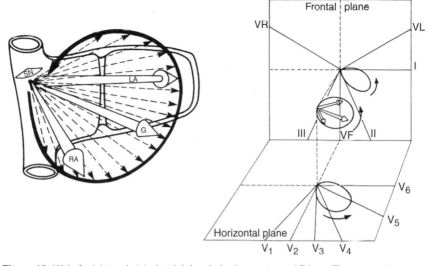

Figure 16 (A) Left, right and global atrial depolarisation vector and P loop. The successive multiple instantaneous vectors are also pictured. (B) P loop and its projection on frontal and horizontal planes.

union of the heads of all atrial depolarisation vectors represents **the P loop**, which is recorded on the ECG as the initial deflection, **the P wave** (Figures 1A, 15 and 16). The loop–hemifield correlation explains the morphology of P wave in different leads (Figure 16). Generally, atrial repolarisation (Ta wave) is seldom seen, being masked by the significant forces generated by ventricular depolarisation that give rise to the QRS complex (Figure 15).

From the end of atrial depolarisation to the beginning of ventricular depolarisation (PR segment in ECG), the electric stimulus depolarises small structures and, therefore, no waves are recorded on the surface ECG (Figure 15) although depolarisation of the bundle of His and its branches can be recorded with intracavitary recording techniques (hisiogram) (Figure 15).

Ventricular depolarisation is carried out in three successive phases that give rise to the generation of three vectors (the expression of three dipoles). Each of the three vectors explains a deflection of the QRS [7]. Ventricular depolarisation begins in three different sites in the left ventricle [8]: areas of the anterior and posterior papillary muscles and a mid-septal area (Figures 17A, C and D); at almost the same time, the right ventricle begins its depolarisation. These three initial depolarisation sites in the left ventricle dominate the small initial forces of the right ventricle and originate a joint depolarisation dipole (vector), which receives the name of **first vector** (Figure 17B). This first vector is directed anteriorly and to the right and, generally, upwards (Figures 18A and B), although in some subjects, especially obese individuals, it may be directed downwards (Figure 18C). Once this initial area in the left ventricle is depolarised, most of the right and left ventricular mass is depolarised at the same time, giving rise

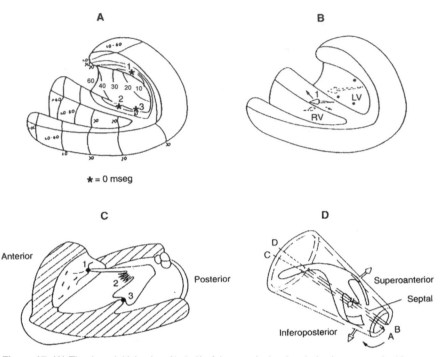

★ = 0 mseg

Figure 17 (A) The three initial points (1, 2, 3) of the ventricular depolarisation are marked by an asterisk (*). The isochronic lines of the depolarisation sequence can also be seen (adapted from Durrer-8). (B) The first vector of the ventricular depolarisation indicated by the continuous line arrow (1) is the result of the sum of the initial depolarisation vectors of the left and right ventricles (dotted arrows). The first vector corresponds to the sum of depolarisation of the three points indicated in (A) and, as it is more potent than the forces of the right vector, the global direction of vector 1 will be from left to right. (C) Left lateral view showing the left papillary muscles and the divisions of the left bundle branch. 1: superoanterior; 2: medioseptal (inconstant); 3: inferoposterior. There is an excellent correlation between the divisions of the left bundle and the three initial points of ventricular depolarisation (1 and 3 always and 2 when present) (A). (D) The superoanterior and inferoposterior divisions in an imaginary left ventricular conus. This is the real position of the division of left bundle in the human heart. The medial fibres on occasions mimic the third fascicle, but appear more often as a net (C).

to a right depolarisation vector (2r) and a left depolarisation vector (2i). The sum of these vectors is directed to the left, somewhat posteriorly and, generally, downwards (Figures 18A and B) and is known as the **second vector**. In obese individuals, it is usually located around 0° (Figure 18C). Finally, the more delayed areas of depolarisation in both ventricles (the areas with fewer Purkinje fibres), i.e. the basal septal areas, originate a **third vector**, which is directed upwards, somewhat to the right and posteriorly (Figure 18). As we have stated, the union of the heads of these three vectors, which is merely a simplification of the union of the heads of all the instantaneous vectors originated during ventricular depolarisation, represents the pathway that the electrical stimulus follows when it depolarises the ventricles and is called **QRS loop**

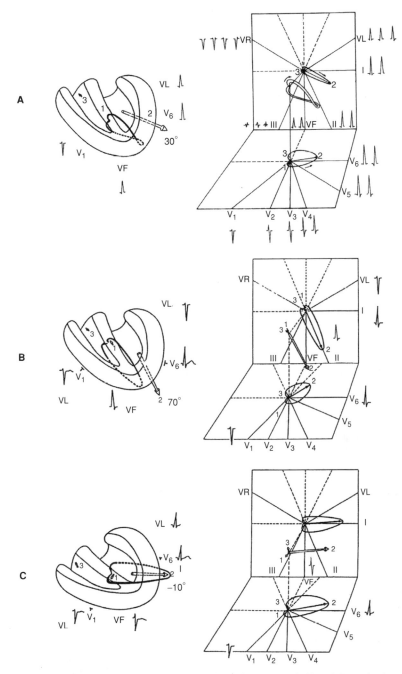

Figure 18 Observe the vectors and ventricular depolarisation loop (left) and the projection of the cardiac vectors and loops on frontal and horizontal planes (right) in a heart with no rotations (A), in the vertical heart (B) (the upward direction of the first vector in A and B is evident) and in the horizontal heart (C) (the first vector is clearly directed downwards).

that originates the **QRS complex in the ECG**) (Figures 1B, 15 and 18). The loop–hemifield correlation explains the morphology of QRS in different leads (Figures 3, 4 and 18).

Finally, ventricular repolarisation takes place, and this also depends mainly on repolarisation of the left ventricular free wall. From a physiological viewpoint, in the subendocardial area there exists a lesser degree of perfusion (physiologic ischaemia) and, as already stated, this explains the positivity in the last part of repolarisation in the leads facing the left ventricle and the negativity in the opposite leads (VR). The pathway that repolarisation follows does not initially show any expression in the ECG and is recorded as an isoelectric ST segment. Later, when a repolarisation dipole is formed, the union of the heads of all instantaneous vectors originates the **T loop** that is recorded as a **T wave in the ECG** (Figures 1C, D and 15).

After the T wave, which represents the end of ventricular systole, and until the beginning of the next atrial systole, an isoelectric line corresponding to the rest phase of all cardiac cells is recorded. Sometimes a small wave, called **U wave**, that forms part of the repolarisation process is recorded after the T wave (Figure 15).

The P, QRS and T loops overall have an orientation that may be expressed by a maximum vector. Although these vectors provide important information on ECG morphology in different leads, only the global contour of the loop, its sense of rotation and the loop–hemifield correlation will explain the total ECG morphology (Figures 1, 3, 14, 16 and 18).

CHAPTER 4

ECG machines: how to perform and interpret ECG

The most common electrocardiographic recording devices used are the direct inscription types with thermosensitive paper (Figure 19). Nowadays, digital recording devices are the most frequently used. Wireless ECG devices are now more and more common. The electrocardiograph records cardiac electric activity conducted through wires to metal plates placed at different points called leads. Wireless ECG devices are now more and more common. The standard 12-lead electrocardiogram (I, II, III, VR, VL, VF and V1–V6) must be performed simultaneously with 3, 6 or 12 leads recorded at the same time, depending on the number of channels of the electrocardiograph. It is convenient that the ECG leads can be displayed and appropriately labelled in their anatomical continuous sequence (VL, I, -VR, II, VF, III see Figure 12). This helps to show any ST deviation in two consecutive leads in cases of acute coronary syndrome (ACS), (see p. 83).

The electric current generated by the heart is conducted through the wires or transmitted wireless by radio to the recording device, which consists fundamentally of an amplifier that magnifies the electric signals and a galvanometer that moves the inscription needle. The needle moves in accordance with the magnitude of the electric potential generated by the patient's heart. This electric potential has a vectorial expression. **The needle inscribes a positive or negative deflection, depending on whether the explorer electrode of a given lead faces the head or the tail of the depolarisation or repolarisation vector** (corresponding to the positive or negative charge of the dipole) regardless of whether or not the electric force is going towards or away from the positive pole of the lead (Figures 9 and 19).

The electrocardiogram (ECG) recording must be performed by trained personnel, though not necessarily by physicians. Prior to interpretation of the ECG, it must be ensured that the recording is correctly done (II = I + III) and that calibration is correct (1 cm = 1 mV) with a smooth slope of the calibration curve. The voltage is usually 1 cm = 1 mV, and recording speed 25 mm/s. In order to better appreciate small changes of ST segment, which is very important in the diagnosis of ACS, it is convenient that ECG recording may be properly amplified.

Interpretation may be manual or automatic. Although modern ECG devices may provide a presumptive diagnosis of encountered ECG abnormalities we should not rely completely on automatically obtained diagnosis alone. What is usually correct is the automatic measurement of different intervals and waves

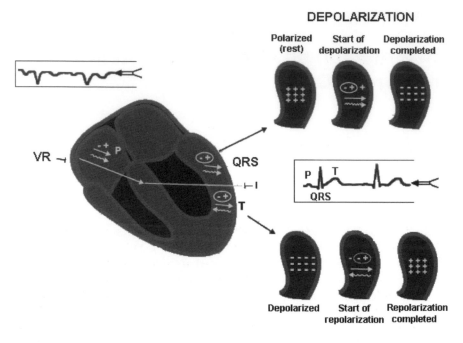

Figure 19 ECG recording from VR and I. Correlation with depolarisation and repolarisation patterns.

(heart rate, PR, P, QRS, OT). However, careful analysis of automatic ECG diagnosis by a physician is always advisable. Furthermore, ECG tracing should be analysed as a whole with the clinical status of a patient. In our opinion, automatic interpretation is especially useful as a screening procedure, particularly in epidemiologic studies.

The manual interpretation has to follow a sequential approach that includes
1 measuring heart rate,
2 knowing the heart rhythm,
3 measuring PR interval and segment and QT interval,
4 calculating the electrical axis of the heart,
5 analysing sequentially the different waves and segments of the ECG (P, QRS, ST, T and U waves).

CHAPTER 5

Normal ECG characteristics

Different items should be routinely assessed when reading an ECG. The names given to different waves and intervals are shown in Figure 15. Different morphologies of P, QRS and T waves have been explained in Figure 2.

Heart rate

Sinus rhythm at rest normally ranges from 60 to 90 beats per minute. Several procedures exist to assess the heart rate on ECG. The graph paper is divided into 5-mm rectangles and, additionally, divided into other smaller rectangles of 1 mm. We may use the following methods to measure the heart rate. (1) Observe the number of 5-mm spaces (when the paper runs at a speed of 25 mm/s, it is equivalent to 0.20 s) between two consecutive R waves. Heart rate assessment according to the R–R interval is shown in Table 1. (2) Observe the RR cycles occurring in 6 s (every five 5-mm space is equal to 1 s) and multiply this number by 10. This is the best method when arrhythmia is present. (3) Use a proper ruler (Figure 20).

Rhythm

This can be normal sinus rhythm or ectopic rhythm. Sinus rhythm is considered according to the loop–hemifield correlation when the P wave is positive in I, II, VF, and from V2 to V6, or positive or ± in III and V1, positive or −/+ in VL and negative in VR. Figure 21 explains, according to rotation of the loop (anticlockwise in sinus rhythm or clockwise in ectopic rhythm), why in normal sinus rhythm P-wave morphology in V1 and III is ± while in atrial ectopic rhythm the morphology of ectopic P wave in V1 and III is −/+. The same correlation is useful to explain the morphologies of P, QRS or T waves seen in other leads. For example, when the axis of the loop is located around +60° the morphology of a sinus P wave in VL will be −/+.

PR interval and segment (Figures 15 and 20)

PR interval is the distance from the beginning of P wave to the beginning of QRS complex (Figure 15A). How this measurement has to be performed is shown in Figure 20. Normal PR interval values in adults range from 0.12 to 0.20 seconds (up to 0.22 seconds in the elderly and even under 0.12 seconds in the newborn). Longer PR intervals are seen in the cases of AV block and

Table 1 Calculation of heart rate according to the RR interval.

Number of 0.20-second spaces	Heart rate
1	300
2	150
3	100
4	75
5	60
6	50
7	43
8	37
9	33

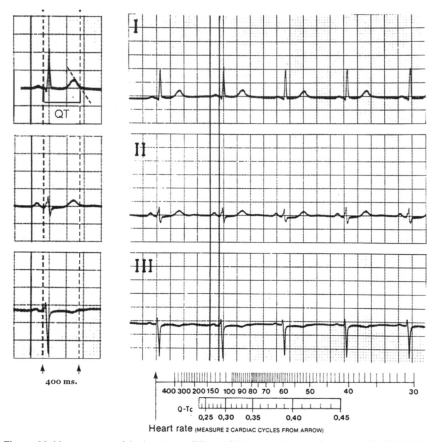

Figure 20 Measurement of the heart rate, PR and QT intervals. In the left one amplified P–QRS–T of leads I, II, III. **Heart rate:** the arrow is located at the onset of the QRS complex. Two cardiac cycles (RR cycles) are measured from the arrow. The distance correlates with the heart rate value on the ruler. In this case, HR is 61 bpm. **PR interval** measured with the three-channel device. The exact PR interval measurement is the longest distance from the earliest onset of the P wave in the given lead (in this case III) to the earliest onset of the QRS complex in any lead (in this case also in III lead). **QT interval measurement:** the QT interval of the first cycle should be measured from the onset of the Q wave to the end of the T wave (400 ms). The corrected QT (QTc) (QT in relation to heart rate) is obtained with a ruler that gives us the result when the end of two RR cycles coincides with the QTc value figuring on the ruler – in this case QTc = 0.39 (390 ms). It is normal if QTc does not exceed, as in this case, the 10–15% of the QTc shown in the ruler (see the text).

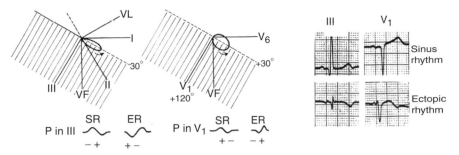

Figure 21 The sinus P wave (anti-clockwise rotation in FP and HP, and ± morphology in III and V1 and −/+ in VL) and ectopic P wave (clockwise rotation and morphology −/+ in III and V1 and ± in VL).

shorter PR intervals in pre-excitation syndromes and different arrhythmias. The PR segment is the distance from the end of P wave to the QRS onset and is usually isoelectric. However, with intracardiac recordings the depolarisation of His bundle may be seen. Figure 15 shows the different spaces of PR interval taken with this technique (see the caption). Sympathetic overdrive may present the descendent PR segment that forms part of an arch of circumference with the ascendent ST segment (Figure 22C). In pericarditis and other diseases affecting the atrial myocardium, as in atrial infarction, a descent or more frequently ascent of PR segment may be seen.

QT interval (Figures 15 and 20)

QT interval represents the sum of depolarisation (QRS complex) and repolarisation (ST segment and T wave). Very often, particularly in the cases of flat T wave or presence of U wave, it is difficult to appropriately measure the QT interval. It is usually considered that this measurement should be performed using a consistent method to ensure that the same measurement is performed if the QT interval is studied sequentially [9]. The most recommended method is to consider the end of repolarisation as a point where the tangent line following the descendent slope of T wave crosses the isoelectric line (Figure 20, left). The best result may be obtained by measuring the median duration of QT in simultaneous 12 leads.

It is necessary to correct the QT interval by the heart rate (QTc). Different heart rate correction formulae exist. The most frequently used are those of the Bazzet and Fredericia. In clinical practice, QTc may be measured with a ruler (Figure 20), and it is considered that its duration should not exceed around 10% of the value corresponding to the heart rate (Figure 20).

A long QT interval may be found in congenital long QT syndrome [10], heart failure, ischaemic heart disease, some electrolyte disorders and following the intake of different drugs. It is considered that a drug should not increase the QTc more than 30 ms and that a change of 60 ms may result in "torsade de pointes' (TdP) occurrence and sudden cardiac death. Nevertheless, TdP rarely occurs unless QTc exceeds 500 ms [9,11]. A **short QT interval** can be found in the cases of early repolarisation, digitalis effect and rarely in some genetic disorders associated with sudden death [12]. Usually in these last cases the QT is shorter than 300 ms.

P wave

This is the atrial depolarisation wave (Figures 1, 15 and 16). In general, its height should not exceed 2.5 mm and its width should not exceed 0.10 seconds. It is rounded and positive but may be ± in V1 and III and −/+ in VL according to the loop–hemifield correlation (Figures 13, 16 and 21).

QRS complex

This corresponds to ventricular depolarisation. Its morphology varies in the different leads according to the loop–hemifield correlation (Figures 1 and 18). An example of this correlation in a heart without rotations (A) and in a heart with vertical (B) and horizontal (C) rotations is shown in Figure 18.

The width should not be less than 0.10 seconds and R-wave height should not exceed 25 mm in leads V5 and V6, or 20 mm in leads I and VL, although in VL the height greater than 15 mm is usually abnormal. Furthermore, the Q wave must be narrow (less than 0.04 seconds) and of quick recording, and does not usually exceed 25% of the following R wave, though some exceptions exist mainly in leads III, VL and VF. Different morphologies are presented in Figure 18. Figure 2 shows the different forms to express the different morphologies of QRS.

ST segment and T wave

The T wave, together with the preceding ST segment, is generated during ventricular repolarisation (Figures 1C and 15). According to the loop–hemifield correlation, in adults, the T wave is positive but with the up-slope slower than the down-slope in all leads, except VR (as the T loop is located in the negative hemifield of that lead). It is usually negative, flattened or occasionally slightly positive in V1, and sometimes may also be flattened or slightly negative in V2, and sometimes even in V3 in women and in Blacks. In III and VF, the T wave may be flattened or even slightly negative. In children, a negative T wave of characteristic morphology seen in the right precordial leads is the normal pattern (children's repolarisation) (Figure 22E).

Under normal conditions, the ST segment is isoelectric (Figure 15) or shows only a small descent slope (<0.5 mm) with ascendent inclination, or a small ascent slope that is convex in relation to the isoelectric line and usually more visible in V1–V2.

Examples of normal ST–T-wave variants are displayed in Figure 22. Let us comment on some of these patterns (see the caption). The saddle-type pattern (Figure 22G) can be observed in V1 in healthy people, especially in subjects with pectus excavatus or when the V1–V2 leads are located in a higher positive (second intercostal space). This pattern should be differentiated from

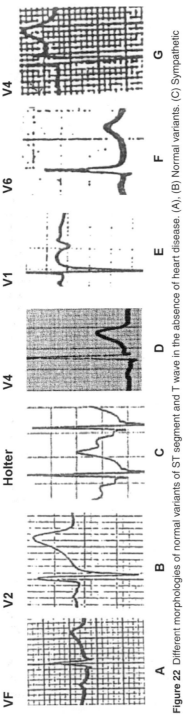
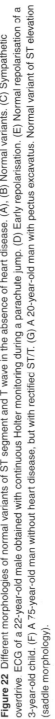

VF   V2

	Holter	V4
A	B	
	C	D

V1   V6   V4

E   F   G

Figure 22 Different morphologies of normal variants of ST segment and T wave in the absence of heart disease. (A), (B) Normal variants. (C) Sympathetic overdrive. ECG of a 22-year-old male obtained with continuous Holter monitoring during a parachute jump. (D) Early repolarisation. (E) Normal repolarisation of a 3-year-old child. (F) A 75-year-old man without heart disease, but with rectified ST/T. (G) A 20-year-old man with pectus excavatus. Normal variant of ST elevation (saddle morphology).

the type-II Brugada pattern (see Figure 105). The pattern of early repolarisation (Figure 22D), ST elevation of even 2–3 mm with downward convexity, is especially recorded in mid-precordial leads. In early repolarisation, the ST-segment elevation normalises with exercise. Acute pericarditis or even an acute coronary syndrome, when ST-segment elevation is seen in the same leads, should be ruled out.

Occasionally, after a T wave, a small wave, called U wave, can be observed usually showing the same polarity as the T wave (Figure 15).

Assessment of the QRS electrical axis in the frontal plane

When the QRS axis is at $+60°$ the morphology in I, II and III is positive but more positive in II according to the rule $II = I + III$ (the same rule may be followed for P- and T-wave-axis assessment) (Figure 23A). When the axis shifts to the left from $+60°$ to $+30°$ etc. up to $-120°$, the QRS complexes become negative starting from lead III, changing from positive to isodiphasic and then from isodiphasic to negative for each shift of $30°$ to the left in the electrical axis (Figures 23A, B and 24A). As the axis shifts to the right from $+60°$ to $90°$ etc., up to $-120°$, complexes again become negative, but starting from lead I, changing from positive to isodiphasic and then from isodiphasic to negative for each $30°$ shift in the electrical axis (Figures 23A, C and 24B). Using this procedure the ÂQRS may be calculated in the frontal plane with a proximity of $30°$. To locate more precisely, the morphology in VR, VL and VF leads needs to be checked. For instance, a positive R wave in I, II and III means that ÂQRS is around $+60°$. If we observe VL, the QRS exactly at $+60°$ is isodiphasic (⌁). According to the loop–hemifield correlation if the complex in VL is more positive than negative, it is located between $+30°$ and $+60°$ and if the QRS complex is more negative than positive the ÂQRS is between $+60°$ and $+90°$.

P, QRS and T electric axis normal values are as follows: (1) ÂP: in more than $90°$ of normal cases, it is located between $+30°$ and $+70°$; (2) ÂQRS: it generally ranges from $0°$ to $+80°$, although it can be located somewhat more to the left in picnics and more to the right in asthenics; (3) ÂT: it generally ranges from $0°$ to $+70°$. ÂT located more to the left occurs when the ÂQRS is also shifted to the left. Nevertheless, with an ÂQRS shifted to the right, on certain occasions ÂT is between $0°$ and $-30°$.

Rotations of the heart

In a heart with no apparent rotation (intermediate position) the ÂQRS is situated around $+30°$. The loop and axis of QRS in a heart with these characteristics are shown in Figure 18A. Nevertheless, the heart may present isolated or combined rotations, the most characteristic of which are rotations on the following axes: the anteroposterior (vertical or horizontal heart; see VL and VF leads in Figures 18B, C and 25) and longitudinal (dextrorotation or levorotation; see precordial leads in Figure 25). Also, a rotation on the transversal axis may be

A

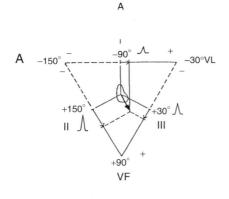

B

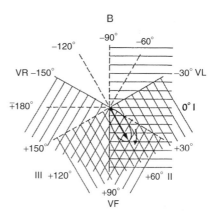

A

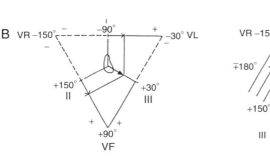

B

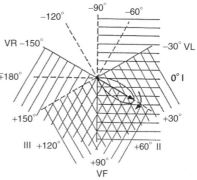

A

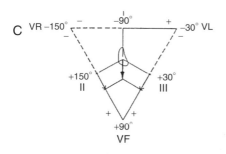

B

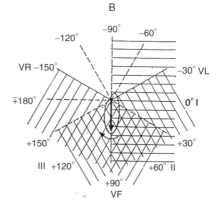

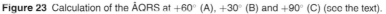

Figure 23 Calculation of the ÂQRS at +60° (A), +30° (B) and +90° (C) (see the text).

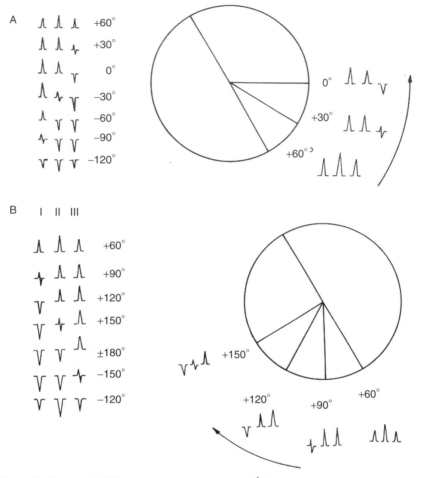

Figure 24 Changes in QRS morphology with 30° shifts of ÂQRS starting from +60° to the left (A) and to the right (B).

seen. In this case, on occasions, the last part of cardiac depolarisation is located upwards and to the right. This explains the pattern S_I S_{II} S_{III} (Figure 43). This pattern may be seen in normal individuals but also in right ventricular hypertrophy and the differential diagnosis with left anterior hemiblock has to be done (Figure 43). Verticalisation is usually associated with dextrorotation (rS in VL, qR in VF and Rs in V6) and horizontalisation with levorotation (qR in VL, rS in VF and RS in V2–V3) (Figure 25). Attention should also be paid to one specific type of combined rotation – dextrorotation with horizontalisation – that occurs due to diaphragm elevation (obesity, pregnancy). This combined rotation explains the morphology with S in lead I, Q in lead III with negative T wave in lead III, which may be confused with inferior myocardial infarction (Figure 26). This QR morphology usually disappears with deep respiration.

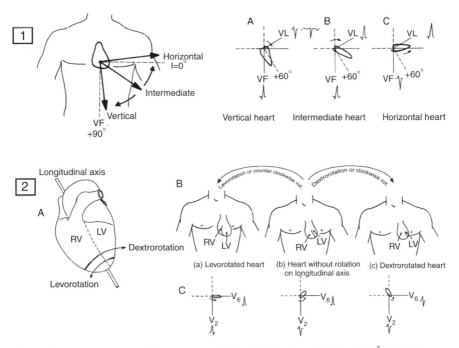

Figure 25 1: Rotation of the heart along the anteroposterior axis. Direction of the ÂQRS in the vertical and horizontal heart. ÂQRS morphology in the vertical (A), intermediate (B) and horizontal heart (C). 2: (A) Rotation of the heart along the longitudinal axis. (B) Scheme of dextrorotation and levorotation. (C) The respective loops and morphologies on the horizontal plane (V2 and V6) in levorotated heart, intermediate heart and dextrorotated heart.

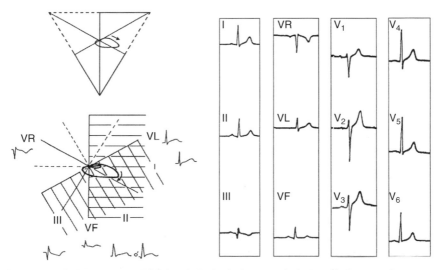

Figure 26 (A) QRS loop and ECG morphologies in the case of a heart with dextrorotation, horizontalisation and apex forward. (B) An example of ECG in a healthy, obese 35-year-old woman with this kind of rotation.

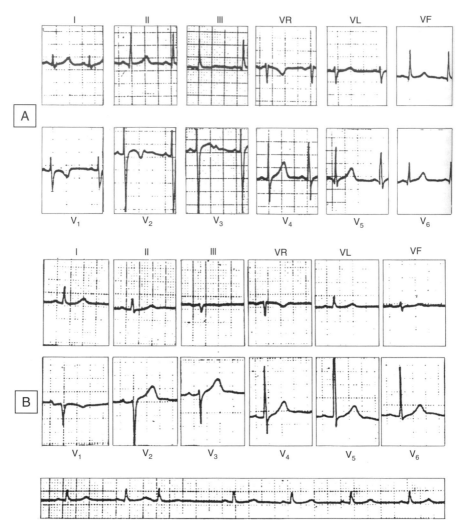

Figure 27 (A) ECG of a 3-year-old child. (B) ECG of an 80-year-old normal man.

Electrocardiographic changes with age (Figure 27)

Infants, children and adolescents (Figure 27A)

The most important features of the ECG of healthy children as compared to normal adults can be summarised as follows:

1 There is a faster heart rate and shorter PR interval.

2 Due to the physiological right ventricular hypertrophy of infants, the heart is usually vertical with ÂQRS to the right and negative or bimodal T waves in V1 to V3–V4, and has a characteristic morphology (infantile repolarisation) that can be seen until adolescence, particularly in females. The QRS loop goes to the left before going back, which explains why the morphology of V6 looks

like the adult's morphology before V1 (there is higher R in V1 compared with 'q' in V6). Sometimes the rsr' pattern is observed in V1. In infants, especially if they are post-term, even R or qR patterns can be seen at birth with a somewhat positive T wave. The Rs pattern persists for a time, perhaps even years even until adulthood. However, the T wave usually becomes flattened or negative in the days following birth.

3 In some adolescents, an R wave with high voltage in precordial leads (Sv2 + RV5 > 60 mm) without the existence of left ventricular enlargement may be seen.

4 Sometimes evident increase in the heart rate with inspiration.

Elderly subjects (Figure 27B)

The following phenomena can be considered age-related variants in ECGs of the elderly:

1 A slower heart rate and longer PR interval (normal until 0.22 seconds).

2 Occasionally, a more right-pointing ÂP is present because of pulmonary emphysema with the 'S' wave in lead V6 and an ÂQRS that, in general, points more to the left (from 0° to −30°).

3 A poor 'r' progression from V1 to V3, probably due to septal fibrosis. This can produce problems in the differential diagnosis with septal necrosis.

4 Some alteration of repolarisation (slightly depressed ST segment and/or flattened T wave). A frequent 'U' wave particularly in the intermediate precordial leads.

CHAPTER 6

Electrocardiographic diagnostic criteria

Electrocardiography can be considered the test of choice, the 'gold standard', for the diagnosis of atrial and ventricular blocks, ventricular pre-excitation, most cardiac arrhythmias and acute myocardial infarction. However, in other cases, such as atrial and ventricular enlargement, abnormalities secondary to chronic coronary artery disease (electrocardiographic pattern of ischaemia or necrosis), in the assessment of other repolarisation abnormalities or certain ar-rhythmias, electrocardiography provides useful information and may suggest the diagnosis based on predetermined **electrocardiographic criteria**; however, these criteria have lesser diagnostic potential compared with other electrocar-diological or imaging techniques (echocardiography, for example, for atrial or ventricular enlargement, etc.). In conditions for which electrocardiography is the technique of choice, the electrocardiographic criteria we use are diagnostic for that disease (e.g. blocks), while for other conditions (e.g. cavity enlarge-ment) the criteria are only indicative of that disease.

Regarding diagnostic criteria employed in electrocardiography (ECG) (or other techniques) when these are not techniques of choice for the diagnosis of a certain condition, e.g. diagnostic ECG criteria for atrial or ventricular enlargement, chronic myocardial infarction, ventricular tachycardia, etc., it is necessary to know their real usefulness. To this end, it is mandatory to apply the concepts of sensitivity, specificity and predictive value.

Specificity of an electrocardiographic criterion (e.g. height of R wave in V5 > 35 mm for left ventricular hypertrophy) is defined as 100 – the percentage of normal individuals that present with that criterion. An electrocardiographic criterion will be more specific when presented by fewer normal individuals. When no normal individuals present these criteria, specificity is 100% (no false positive cases will be found).

$$\text{Specificity} = \frac{\text{True negatives (TN)}}{\text{TN} + \text{False positives (FP)}} \times 100$$

Sensitivity of an electrocardiographic criterion (e.g. height of R wave in V5 > 35 mm for left ventricular hypertrophy) is defined as 100 – the percentage of individuals with a determined abnormality (in this case left ventricular hypertrophy) presenting with that criterion. If all the individuals with the heart disease under discussion show a certain electrocardiographic criterion, the sensitivity will be 100% (no false negative cases will be found).

$$\text{Sensitivity} = \frac{\text{True positive (TP)}}{\text{TP} + \text{False negatives (FN)}} \times 100$$

As can be appreciated, specificity is determined in a control group (patients without the abnormality under study) and sensitivity in a group with the abnormality once other first-choice techniques (echocardiography, angiography, etc.) have been used to define these two groups with or without the abnormality under study.

Predictive value represents the clinical significance of a criterion. It indicates the probability of a result being valid, bearing in mind the concrete result of the criterion, whether positive or negative. It signifies what is the percentage of patients with a criterion who will suffer from that disease (f.i. percentage of valvular heart disease patients with P± in II, III and VF that will present left atrial enlargement – **positive predictive value**) or what is the percentage of patients without the criterion under discussion who do not suffer that disease (**negative predictive value**).

$$PPV = \frac{TP}{TP + FP} \qquad NPV = \frac{TN}{TN + FN}$$

The predictive value of an ECG criterion (f.i. P± in II, III, VF) to predict left atrial enlargement in patients with valve heart disease must be assessed on the basis of the epidemiological reality because it is related to the prevalence of the ECG criterion in the population studied. This means that we need to study a consecutive group of patients, in this case, with valve heart disease, to know the predictive value of this ECG criterion to detect left atrial enlargement already proven by echocardiography. Therefore, we cannot use, to know the predictive value (for positives and negatives), the sample sizes chosen at random to assess sensitivity and especificity of the same criterion (e.g. 100 patients with and 100 without left atrial enlargement detected by echocardiography), unless the corrections that are appropriate for the epidemiological reality are applied. Table 2 shows the practical form to detect sensitivity, specificity and predictive

Table 2 Calculation of sensitivity (SE), specificity (SP), positive and negative predictive values (PPV, NPV) of a certain electrocardiographic criterion.

100 VALVULAR PATIENTS				
		LAE by echocardiography		
		YES	NO	Total
100 Valvular patients	P± en II, III, VF	2	0	2	$PPV = \dfrac{TP}{TP + FP} = \dfrac{2}{2 + 0} \times 100 \approx 100\%$
	Without p± en II, III, VF	88	10	98	$NPV = \dfrac{TN}{TN + FN} = \dfrac{10}{10 + 88} \times 100 \approx 10\%$
Total		90	10	100	
$SE \dfrac{TP}{TP + FN} = \dfrac{2}{2 + 88} \times 100 \approx 2\%$			$SP \dfrac{TN}{TN + FP} = \dfrac{10}{10 + 0} \times 100 = 100\%$	

An example to demonstrate whether the presence of an electrocardiographic criterion (in this case a +/− P wave in II, III and aVF in patients with valvular heart disease) does or does not predict the presence of left atrial enlargement (LAE) as detected by echocardiography.

Abbreviations: PPV, positive predictive value; NPV, negative predictive value; TP, true positive; FP, false positive; TN, true negative; FN, false negative; SE, sensitivity; SP, specificity.

value taking as an example the criterion of left atrial enlargement (LAE) P ± in II, III, VF in a group of 100 patients with valvular heart disease. We use the table 2 × 2 (Table 2). All cases have an echocardiogram as a gold standard for LAE. The cases with P ± in II, III, VF are located in the upper part of the table, and the cases that do not present this ECG criterion in the lower part. In both rows there are cases with and without LAE by echocardiography. The table shows how easily we may perform the calculation of SP, SE, PPV and NPV using the formulae explained earlier. It is important to remember that for calculation of PV (positive and negative) we have to consider the epidemiological reality and we have to study a cohort of consecutive patients.

It must be borne in mind that sensitivity and specificity of different electro-cardiographic criteria vary in an inverse manner, so that very specific criteria will not be very sensitive (e.g. P wave > 0.15 seconds or with ± morphology in II, III, VF is very specific criterion for the diagnosis of left atrial enlargement (LAE), as a very small number of patients without LAE will present it; however, it is not very sensitive, as few patients with LAE have a P wave with that duration or morphology). Given this inverse relationship, it is difficult to find criteria that maintain a high level of sensitivity without losing specificity.

Finally, it should be stated that the accuracy of an electrocardiographic criterion or test increases, according to Bayes' theorem, when applied to a population with a high prevalence of a given heart disease (high a priori probability of having the disease) and decreases when applied to a population with a low prevalence of that heart disease (low a priori probability). Thus, the value of ST-segment depression as a criterion of coronary heart disease is much higher if found in a population with a high prevalence of coronary heart disease (middle-aged patient with family history, chest pain and risk factors (hyperc-holesterolemia, high blood pressure, diabetes)) than in a population with a low prevalence of coronary heart disease (e.g. young adults with no risk factors).

CHAPTER 7

Atrial abnormalities

All the electrocardiographic patterns observed in patients with atrial enlargement and with atrial conduction blocks are encompassed by this term (Figures
28–30). It is convenient to bear in mind the following facts [1]:

1 The normal P wave (Figures 16, 28A and 29A) is explained by activation first
of the right atrium and then of the left atrium, with an intermediate period
during which both atria are depolarised together [13,14].

2 Atria become dilated more than hypertrophied.

3 The classical morphology of P wave in right atrial enlargement is an increase
in voltage without increase in length (Figures 28B, 29B and C).

4 The classical morphology of left atrial enlargement is secondary to the delay
in interatrial conduction rather than to atrial dilation (Figures 28C and 29D)
[15].

5 P-wave voltage is influenced by extracardiac factors that increase (hypoxia,
sympathicotonia, etc.) or decrease it (emphysema, atrial fibrosis, etc.).

6 In an interatrial block, the conduction delay occurs between the right and
left atria. Although usually associated with left atrial enlargement, it may also
exist as an isolated finding in the cases of pericarditis, ischaemic heart disease,
etc. The block can be partial or complete.

Right atrial enlargement (Figures 28B, 29B and C)

Right atrial enlargement (RAE) is especially present in patients with congenital
and valvular heart diseases affecting the right side of the heart and in cor
pulmonale.

Diagnostic criteria
Diagnostic criteria of RAE are based on the following:

1 QRS complex alterations: (1) 'qr (qR)' morphology in V1 in the absence of
an infarction (specificity = 100% according to some authors); (2) QRS complex
voltage ≤4 mm in V1 and V2/V1 QRS complex voltage ≥5 (quite a specific
criterion, SP = 90%).

2 P-wave abnormalities (P ≥ 2.5 mm in II and/or 1.5 mm in V1). These criteria
have low sensitivity and they are somewhat more specific.

Left atrial enlargement (Figures 28C and 29D)

Left atrial enlargement (LAE) is seen in patients with mitral and aortic valvular
disease, ischaemic heart disease, hypertension and some cardiomyopathies.

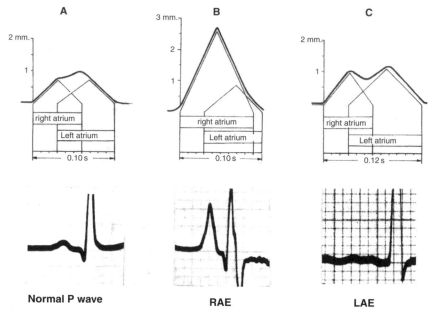

Figure 28 Top: scheme of atrial depolarisation in (A) normal P wave, (B) right atrial enlargement (RAE) and (C) left atrial enlargement (LAE). Bottom: three examples of these P waves.

Diagnostic criteria

The diagnostic criteria of LAE are as follows:

1 P wave with a duration ≥0.12 seconds especially seen in leads I or II, generally bimodal, but with normal height.

2 Diphasic P wave in V1 with an evident final negativity of at least 0.04 seconds because the second part of the loop is directed backwards due to left atrial enlargement (see Figure 29D – HP).

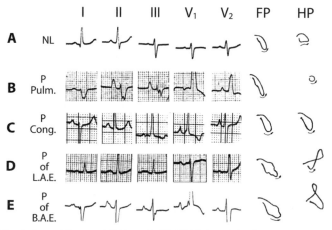

Figure 29 Morphology of P wave. (A) Normal. (B), (C) Right atrial enlargement: (B) P pulmonale; (C) P congenitale; (D) left atrial enlargement (P mitrale); and (E) biatrial enlargement.

These two criteria have a good specificity (close to 90%) (few false positive cases), but a discrete sensitivity (lower than 60%) (more false negative cases).
1 The ± P-wave morphology in II, III and VF with P ≥ 0.12 seconds is very specific and presents high PPV (100% in valvular heart disease and cardiomyopathies), though with a low sensitivity and low negative predictive value for left atrial enlargement [16,17] (see Table 2).

Biatrial enlargement (Figure 29E)

Diagnostic criteria

Diagnostic criteria of biatrial enlargement include criteria of right and left atrial enlargement:
1 P wave in II taller (≥2.5 mm) and wider (≥0.12 seconds) than normal. On certain occasions there can be a 'peaked' positive P wave in V1–V2.
2 Criteria of left atrial enlargement with an ÂP shifted to the right and/or criteria of right atrial enlargement based on QRS complex alterations.

Interatrial block*

Partial block

In a partial interatrial block, the stimulus reaches the left atrium via the normal pathway, but with a certain delay.

Diagnostic criteria

P wave with a duration ≥0.12 seconds in the frontal plane. The P-wave length and consequently the bimodal morphology of P wave seen in lead II as a most typical lead detected in an isolated partial interatrial block is similar to the P wave of left atrial enlargement. In fact, as we have already stated, the delay in interatrial conduction, more than left atrium dilation, generally explains the morphology of left atrial enlargement (LAE). However, the morphology of P wave in HP especially V1 is usually different. In the case of an isolated interatrial block (f.i. pericarditis) the second part of the loop is not directed so much backwards because there is no LAE and, consequently, the P wave morphology in V1 is positive or presents only a small negative part.

---

*The concept of a block means that in a certain part of the heart (sinoatrial union, atria, atrioventricular union or ventricles) the electrical stimulus encounters overall significant difficulties for its conduction. If conduction is slow, but the stimulus passes through the area with slow conduction, we call it a first-degree or partial block; when the stimulus is completely blocked we call it a third-degree or complete block, and when the stimulus sometimes passes and sometimes not, we call it a second-degree block.

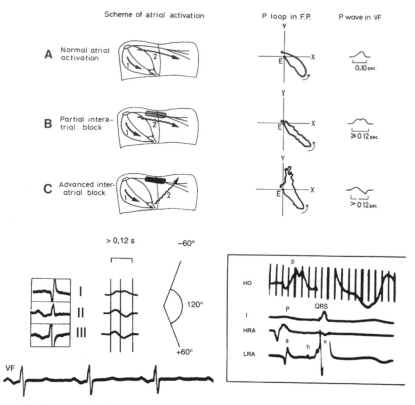

Figure 30 Top: example of atrial activation and characteristics of the P loop in the frontal plane and the morphology of P wave in VF in normal conditions (A), and in the case of partial (B) and complete interatrial block with left atrial retrograde activation (C). Bottom left: leads I, II and III in complete interatrial block with left atrial retrograde activation, with direction of the activation vectors of the first and the second part of the P wave and four consecutive P waves with ± morphology in VF in a patient with complete interatrial block. Bottom right: oesophageal and intracavitary recordings demonstrating the sequence of activation in this type of interatrial block (high right atrium, low right atrium, high oesophageal lead with −/+ morphology).

Complete interatrial block, with left atrial retrograde activation
[16–18] (Figure 30)
In a complete interatrial block, the stimulus does not reach the left atrium via the normal path, but by retrograde left atrial activation [16].

Diagnostic criteria
P wave with a duration ≥0.12 seconds and ± in II, III and VF. P wave ± in V1 to V3–V4 is frequent. This type of block is frequently accompanied by supraventricular arrhythmias, particularly atypical atrial flutter [17,18].

CHAPTER 8

Ventricular enlargement

The electrocardiographic concept of enlargement of right and left ventricles encompasses both hypertrophy and dilatation and, of course, the combination of both processes.

Ventricular enlargement (VE) morphologies are secondary to hypertrophy rather than to dilatation, unlike what occurs in the atria. A certain degree of homolateral block to the enlarged ventricle and interstitial fibrosis are present. As the degree of septal interstitial fibrosis increases, less 'Q' wave is visible in the leads facing the left ventricle such as V5–V6 [19]. Furthermore, the finding of a more or less abnormal ECG recording is related more to the evolutionary phase than to the severity of disease. On the other hand, slight or even moderate degrees of enlargement of either of the ventricles, mainly the right, or of both at the same time, may not produce abnormalities in the ECG.

More than 50 years ago, the Mexican school [20] coined the electrocardiographic concept of systolic and diastolic overload (rSR' in V1 in diastolic overload in right ventricular enlargement as in atrial septal defect and qR with a tall T wave in V5–V6 in the cases of diastolic overload of the left ventricle as in aortic regurgitation) and systolic overload pattern (R waves with the 'strain' pattern of repolarisation-downsloping ST with a negative asymmetrical T wave – recorded in V1–V2 in the case of systolic right ventricle overload as in severe pulmonary stenosis or in V5–V6 in the case of left ventricle systolic overload as aortic stenosis). These concepts later became the subject of great debate. It is currently considered that, regardless of the type of underlying haemodynamic overload, the so-called electrocardiographic pattern of diastolic overload usually corresponds to slight or moderate degrees of right or left ventricular enlargement, while the systolic overload pattern – *strain pattern* – is usually found in very advanced stages of any right or left ventricular enlargement.

The superiority of echocardiography over electrocardiography for the diagnosis of ventricular enlargement, mainly of the left ventricle, is evident (sensitivity is much higher with nearly similar specificity). However, when the ventricular enlargement is diagnosed with the electrocardiogram, the value of the latter is greater than that of the echocardiogram in predicting heart disease evolution and prognosis.

We will address the diagnostic criteria of ventricular enlargement in the cases of QRS duration under 120 ms. For the diagnosis of right and/or left ventricular enlargement combined with ventricular block (QRS duration over 120 ms), we suggest the consultation of other publications [1,5,21,22].

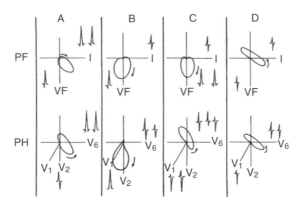

Figure 31 Four different characteristic types of the loop observed in right ventricular enlargement (RVE). (A) Normal frontal plane (FP) and horizontal plane (HP) with the loop directed more anteriorly. This explains the morphology of RS in V1–V2. It is often seen in patients with mitral stenosis and corresponds to a mild RVE. (B) FP with the maximum vector to the right (QRS-type S_I, R_{II}, R_{III}) and HP with the loop directed totally anteriorly and with a clockwise rotation. This corresponds to a severe RVE and is particularly observed in patients with congenital heart diseases or severe pulmonary hypertension. In less-advanced phases of disease the morphology of the QRS loop in HP is somewhat different, e.g. a figure-of-eight morphology. (C) FP with the maximum vector directed to the right (QRS type S_I, R_{II}, R_{III}) and HP with the major part of the loop directed posteriorly and to the right, which usually corresponds to a moderate or even important RVE, and may be seen in patients with chronic cor pulmonale. (D) The loop in HP is similar to the previous one, but with S_I, S_{II}, S_{III} morphology in FP. It is usually seen in moderate–severe RVE.

Right ventricular enlargement

Right ventricular enlargement (RVE) is found particularly in the cases of congenital heart diseases, valvular heart diseases and cor pulmonale. Figures 31 and 32 show the changes that RVE may produce in ventricular loops and how these changes may explain the different ECG patterns. The changes produced move the loop rightwards and posteriorly more as a consequence of the delay of activation of RV than of an increase of right ventricle mass that also exists, but usually is not more important than the mass of left ventricle. The lower part of Figure 31 shows that ECG pattern in V1 (with more or less R wave) is related more to RVE degree than to RVE aetiology.

Diagnostic criteria

The electrocardiographic criteria most frequently used for the diagnosis of right ventricular enlargement are shown in Table 3, along with their sensitivity, which is low, and specificity, which is high. The differential diagnosis of exclusive or predominant R wave in V1 (R, Rs or rSR′ pattern) is shown in Table 4.

1 Morphology of V1. Morphologies with dominant or exclusive R wave in V1 are very specific, but not so sensitive (<10%) for the diagnosis of RVE, since the loop that gives rise to them (anterior and to the right) (Figure 32B–D) is

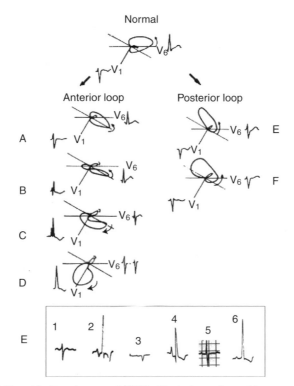

Figure 32 In right ventricular enlargement (RVE) with electrocardiographic repercussion, the horizontal loop of the QRS is always directed to the right, either forwards or backwards. When it is directed forwards, different morphologies may be recorded (from A to D cases with more advanced degree of RVE). A patient may have a morphology changing from one to another during the course of the disease. However, in general, heart diseases with mild to moderate RVE present type A or type B morphologies and those with important RVE present type D. If the loop is directed posteriorly, the morphologies are of types E or F. The QS morphology is seen in the V1 lead in type E, while rS or rSr′ in type F, in both cases accompanied by a significant S in V6. Lower part of the figure shows that the morphology of QRS in V1 depends more on the severity of RVE than on the etiology of the disease. 1, 3 and 5 represent examples of mild mitral stenosis, cor pulmonale and congenital pulmonary stenosis, respectively, while 2, 4 and 6 are the cases of severe and longstanding mitral stenosis, cor pulmonale with severe pulmonary hypertension and congenital pulmonary stenosis, respectively.

observed in a small number of cases with RVE (specially congenital heart disease with systolic overload). In these cases the repolarization present depressed ST with negative and asymetric T wave – strain pattern (Figures 32, 34 and 36) – except in the newborn, which may present exclusive R wave with a positive T wave (see Case 10, p. 139). Nevertheless, other causes that may present a dominant R pattern in V1 must be ruled out (see Table 4). The rS or even QS morphology in V1, but with RS in V6, may often be observed in chronic cor pulmonale, even in advanced phases or in the early phases of RVE of other

Table 3 Electrocardiographic criteria of right ventricular enlargement.

	Criterion	Sensitivity (%)	Specificity (%)
V1	R/S V1 $\geq$ 1	6	98
	R V1 $\geq$ 7 mm	2	99
	qR in V1	5	99
	S in V1 < 2 mm	6	98
	IDT in V1 $\geq$ 0.35 s	8	98
V5–V6	R/S V5–V6 $\leq$ 1	16	93
	R V5–V6 < 5 mm	13	87
	S V5–V6 $\geq$ 7 mm	26	90
V1 + V6	RV1 + SV5–V6 > 10.5 mm	18	94
ÂQRS	ÂQRS $\geq$ 110°	15	96
	S_I, S_{II}, S_{III}	24	87

IDT, intrinsicoid deflection (time from QRS onset to R-wave peak).

Table 4 Morphologies with dominant R or (r′) R′ in V1. Clinical setting, typical morphologies in V1, QRS width, and morphology of P in V1.

Clinical setting	Morphology in V1 with dominant R or R′	QRS width	P-wave morphology in V1
1 No heart disease			
• Incorrect electrodes placement		< 0.12 s	Negative in second ICS and positive or +/− in fourth ICS
• Normal variant (post-term infants, scant Purkinje fibres in anteroseptal zone		< 0.12 s	Normal
• Chest anomalies		< 0.12 s	Normal
2 Typical right bundle branch block		From < 0.12 to $\geq$ 0.12 s	Normal
3 A typical right bundle branch block			
• Ebstein's disease		Often $\geq$ 0.12 s	Often tall and peaked and + or $\pm$
• Arrhythmogenic right ventricular dysplasia		Often $\geq$ 0.12 s	Often abnormal
• Brugada's syndrome		Sometimes $\geq$ 0.12 s	Normal
4 Right ventricular or biventricular enlargement		< 0.12 s	Often tall and peaked
5 WPW syndrome		From < 0.12 to $\geq$ 0.12 s	Normal P, short PR
6 Lateral myocardial infarction		< 0.12 s	Normal P

ICS, intercostal space.

A   B

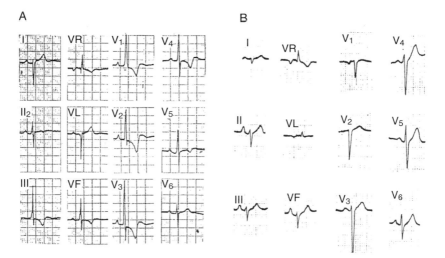

Figure 33 (A) An 8-year-old patient with important pulmonary valve stenosis, with a gradient over 100 mHg. The patient presents a typical morphology of RVE with R-wave-type systolic overload (strain) from V1 to V3. (B) Patient with right ventricular enlargement due to an advanced chronic obstructive pulmonary disease with posterior and right QRS-loop-type S_I, SI_{II}, S_{III}.

aetiologies (Figures 32E and F). The presence of rsR' is especially typical of an atrial septal defect, and in the cases of severe pulmonary stenosis, the most frequent morphology in V1 is a striking R wave with a strain pattern (negative ST/T wave) with the same morphology in V2 (Figure 33A). On the contrary, in cases of pulmonary stenosis of tetralogy of Fallot type, the morphology in V1 is similar to that in isolated pulmonary stenosis, but in V2 this is an rS morphology.

2 Morphology of V6. The presence of evident forces directed to the right expressed as an evident S wave in V5–V6 is one of the most important ECG criteria (see Figures 31 and 32 and Table 3).

3 Electrical axis: ÂQRS $\geq$ + 110°. Inferoposterior hemiblock, vertical heart and lateral infarction must be ruled out. This criterion is quite specific (>95%), but presents low sensitivity. An ÂQRS extremely deviated to the right might suggest RVE due to congenital heart disease (pulmonary stenosis) (Figure 33A). A right ÂQRS usually not more than +90° or +100° may also be seen in chronic obstructive pulmonary disease, but in this case usually the voltage of QRS is lower.

4 S_I, S_{II}, S_{III}. This morphology is frequently seen in chronic cor pulmonale with a QS pattern in V1 and an RS pattern in V6, and represents a sign of bad prognosis (Figure 33B). The possibility of this pattern being secondary to a positional change (p. 29) or simply to the peripheral right ventricular block must be ruled out.

The combination of more than one of these criteria increases the diagnostic possibilities. Horan and Flowers [22] published a scoring system based on the most frequently used ventricular enlargement electrocardiographic criteria.

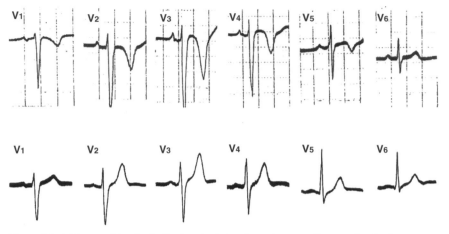

Figure 34 A 60-year-old patient with chronic obstructive pulmonary disease who due to a respiratory infection presented with an electrocardiographic finding of an acute overload pattern of the right chamber (A), which disappeared in a few days (B). Note the change in P- and T-wave morphologies and the disappearance of rS morphology that was observed till V5 as a sign of right ventricular dilation.

Electrocardiographic signs of right acute overload
(Figures 34 and 35)

The electrocardiographic signs more indicative of right acute overload (decompensation of cor pulmonale cor pulmonary embolism) are as follows:

A Change in the ÂQRS (more than 30° to the right of its usual position).
B Transient negative T waves sometimes very evident in right precordial leads (Figure 34).
C S_1, Q_{III} with a negative T_{III} pattern (McGinn and White pattern) in the frontal plane and an RS or rS pattern in V6.
D Appearance of complete right bundle branch block morphology often with ST-segment elevation. The latter two criteria are highly specific but little sensitive for important pulmonary embolism (Figure 35). Nevertheless, the clinical setting and the comparison with previous ECG are very important for a differential diagnosis of both processes to be made.

Left ventricular enlargement

Left ventricular enlargement (LVE) is found particularly in hypertension, ischaemic heart disease, valvular heart disease, cardiomyopathies and some congenital heart diseases.

In general, in patients with left ventricular enlargement, the maximum QRS vector of the loop increases its voltage and is directed more posteriorly than normal (Figure 36). This explains why negativity of QRS predominates in the right

A　　　　　　　　　　B

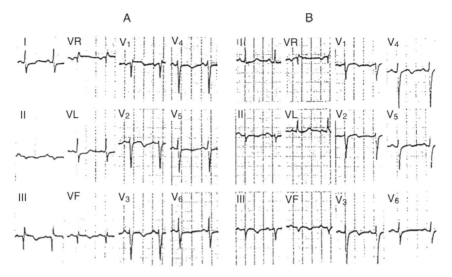

Figure 35 A 59-year-old patient presenting a typical pattern of McGinn and White (SI QIII with negative T wave in lead III) (A) in the course of a pulmonary embolism. (B) The ECG findings after the recovery of the patient.

precordial leads (Figures 36A–C). Occasionally, probably related to significant cardiac levorotation or due to more significant hypertrophy of the left ventricular septal area, than of the left ventricular free wall, as occurs in some cases of apical hypertrophic cardiomyopathy, the maximum vector is not directed posteriorly (it is located close to 0°). This implies a tall R wave that is seen even in V2 (Figure 36E). The presence of striking signs suggestive of left ventricular enlargement (high voltage of QRS + inverted ST-T wave − strain pattern) in an asymptomatic patient without heart murmur or hypertension, suggests hypertrophic cardiomyopathy. In the bottom part of Figure 36 there is the case of aortic valvular disease (left) without fibrosis (q in V6) and a positive T wave, and another (right) with fibrosis (no q wave in V6) and a strain pattern.

The ECG pattern changes during disease evolution. The pattern of 'strain' appears more in relation with the duration of the disease than with the presence of different types of haemodynamic overload. In the past, it was considered that it appears more in the cases of systolic overload (aortic stenosis) than of diastolic overload (aortic regurgitation) [6]. However, a 'q' wave in V5–V6 remains more frequently in long-standing aortic regurgitation than in aortic stenosis (Figure 37). The disappearance of q wave in V6 is probably more related to interstitial septal fibrosis, a substrate of partial left bundle block, than to haemodynamic overload [19] (Figure 36 bottom and Figure 37).

The LVE pattern is usually fixed but may, at least, partially be resolved with medical treatment, as occurs in hypertension (Figure 38) or surgery (valvular heart disease).

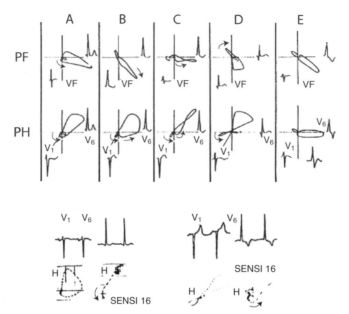

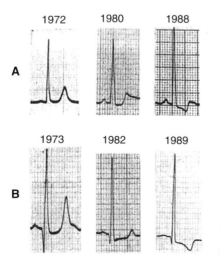

Figure 36 The most characteristic loops of left ventricular enlargement (LVE). (A) With the initial forces to the right and a positive T wave; observed in the cases of LVE that is not long-standing, and with mild septal fibrosis. (B and C) QRS loops initially to the left and with anti-clockwise rotation or figure-of-eight rotation on the horizontal plane; corresponds to significant LVE seen in advanced heart diseases with significant septal fibrosis. (D) QRS loop with 'q' of pseudonecrosis that occurs in some cases of hypertrophic cardiomyopathy with asymmetric septal hypertrophy. (E) QRS loop pointed approximately 0° on the horizontal plane with a very peaked T loop pointed backwards and above characteristic for the apical type of hypertrophic cardiomyopathy. Below: two examples of aortic valve disease; one (left) with mild septal fibrosis and normal ECG and VCG (presence of 'q wave' in V6 as the expression of first vector); the other (right) with important septal fibrosis and abnormal ECG (ST/T with a strain pattern) and VCG (absence of 'q' wave in V6).

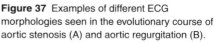

Figure 37 Examples of different ECG morphologies seen in the evolutionary course of aortic stenosis (A) and aortic regurgitation (B).

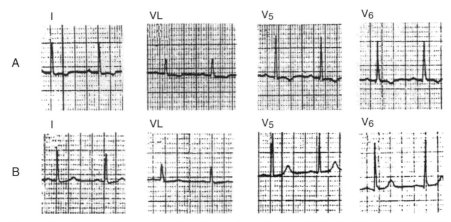

Figure 38 A 56-year-old male with a hypertensive heart disease. ECG before treatment (A) and 7 months later (B). Note that the repolarisation abnormalities of left ventricular enlargement have disappeared.

Diagnostic criteria

Various diagnostic criteria exist (Table 5). Those with good specificity ($\geq$85%) and acceptable sensitivity (between 40% and 55%) include Cornell's voltage criteria and the Rohmilt and Estes scoring system. These diagnostic criteria have many limitations, which are in part secondary to the fact that their usefulness differs according to the population group in which they are employed. According to the Bayes theorem, the possibility that ECG may be useful to diagnose left ventricular enlargement is quite high in a group of severely hypertensive patients and low in an asymptomatic normotensive adults. In hypertensive patients, the value of ECG diagnosic criteria shown in Table 5 is still lower. For these patients the criterion described by Rodriguez Padial [1] is useful, that is the sum of QRS voltage of 12 ECG leads >120 ms.

Table 5 Electrocardiographic criteria of left ventricular enlargement.

Voltage criteria	Sensitivity (%)	Specificity (%)
1 RI + S_{III} > 25 mm	10.6	100
2 RVL > 11 mm	11	100
3 RVL > 7.5 mm	22	96
4 SV1 + RV5–V6 $\geq$ 35 mm (Sokolow–Lyon)	22	100
5 RV5–V6 > 26 mm	25	98
6 RVL + SV3 > 28 mm (men) or 20 mm (women)	42	96
(Cornell voltage criterion)		
7 Cornell voltage duration measurement	51	95
QRS duration × Cornell voltage > 2436 mm/seg		
8 In V1–V6, the deepest S + the tallest R > 45 mm	45	93
9 Romhilt–Estes score > 4 points	55	85
10 Romhilt–Estes score > 5 points	35	95

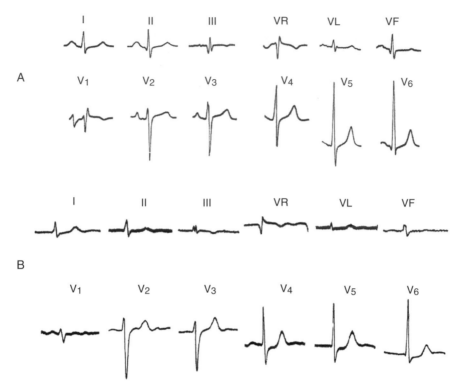

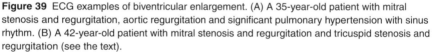

Figure 39 ECG examples of biventricular enlargement. (A) A 35-year-old patient with mitral stenosis and regurgitation, aortic regurgitation and significant pulmonary hypertension with sinus rhythm. (B) A 42-year-old patient with mitral stenosis and regurgitation and tricuspid stenosis and regurgitation (see the text).

Biventricular enlargement (Figure 39)

The electrocardiographic diagnosis of biventricular enlargement is even more difficult than that of isolated enlargement of just one ventricle, as the increased opposing forces of both ventricles often counterbalance themselves or the notable predominance of one ventricle's enlargement masks completely the enlargement of the other.

Diagnostic criteria

The following electrocardiographic criteria suggest the diagnosis of biventricular enlargement:

1 Tall R wave in V5, V6 with an ÂQRS shifted to the right ($\geq 90°$). The presence of an inferoposterior hemiblock associated with left ventricular enlargement as well as asthenic body-build must be ruled out.

2 Tall R wave with 's' in V5, V6 and with an rSR' pattern in V1 and P wave of biatrial enlargement (Figure 39A).

3 QRS complexes within normal limits, but with significant repolarisation abnormalities (negative T wave and depression of ST segment), mainly when the patient presents atrial fibrillation. This type of ECG can be found in the elderly with advanced heart diseases and biventricular enlargement.

4 Small S wave in V1 with a deep S wave in V2 and predominant R wave in V5 and V6 together with an ÂQRS shifted to the right in the frontal plane or an S_I-, S_{II}-, S_{III}-type morphology (Figure 39B).

5 Large voltages in intermediate precordial leads, with tall R waves in the left precordial leads (a frequent finding in patients with ventricular septal defects). It is explained by the existence of a wide and rounded QRS loop in the frontal plane with its final portion directed to the right.

CHAPTER 9

Ventricular blocks

Ventricular conduction disturbances or blocks (Figures 40–47) can occur on the right side (Table 6) or on the left side (Table 7). They can affect the entire ventricle (**global block**) or only part of it (**zonal or divisional block**) and, as explained in Chapter 7, section 'Interatrial block', the block of stimuli in all parts of the heart may be of **first degree (partial block)** when the stimulus passes through the area but with delay, **third degree (complete block)** when passage of stimulus is completely blocked, and **second degree** when the stimulus sometimes passes and sometimes does not. This type of block is known as **aberrancy of conduction**.

The blocked area, wherever it is, is depolarised with certain delay and, in the cases of **complete global** block, depolarises the latest.

Global ventricular block usually shows the stimulus conduction delay in the proximal part of the right or left branches, which is why the ventricular block of global type **is known as bundle branch block.**

Complete or third degree bundle branch block, both right and left, has the following characteristics [7]:

1 Diagnosis is mainly based on data provided by the horizontal plane leads V1 and V6 and the frontal plane lead, VR.

2 The QRS complex must be of at least 0.12 seconds.

3 The slurrings on the QRS are usually opposed to the T wave.

4 Depolarisation of the ventricle corresponding to the blocked branch occurs transseptally, beginning at the contralateral ventricle. This phenomenon explains the QRS complex widening due to the presence of poor Purkinje fibres in the septum and the peculiar QRS complex morphology, both in right and left bundle branch blocks due to the loop–hemifield correlation (Figures 40 and 42).

5 Septal repolarisation dominates over that of the left ventricular free wall and is responsible for the ST–T changes.

6 In general, the anatomical changes are more diffuse than the electrocardiographic expression [23].

Cases with partial bundle branch block (Figure 41) present a QRS less than 120 ms, which gives rise to morphologies sometimes indistinguishable from some patterns seen in the case of homolateral ventricular enlargements (see Figure 32B).

Zonal or divisional left blocks (hemiblocks) [24] have been studied in more depth, both from an anatomical and an electrophysiological viewpoint, compared with right zonal blocks. The latter will only be mentioned in this chapter (Table 6).

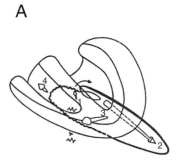

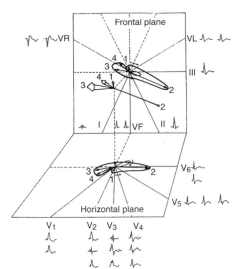

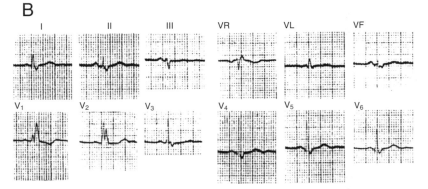

Figure 40 (A) An example of how activation occurs in a complete right bundle branch block and how the different lead morphologies are explained with the loop–hemifield correlation. (B) A typical ECG of a complete right bundle branch block.

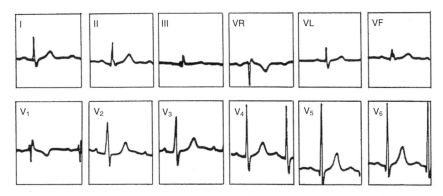

Figure 41 An example of ECG in a partial right bundle branch block. Observe that QRS is less than 0.12 seconds with rSR′ morphology in V1, Qr in VR and qRs in the V6 lead.

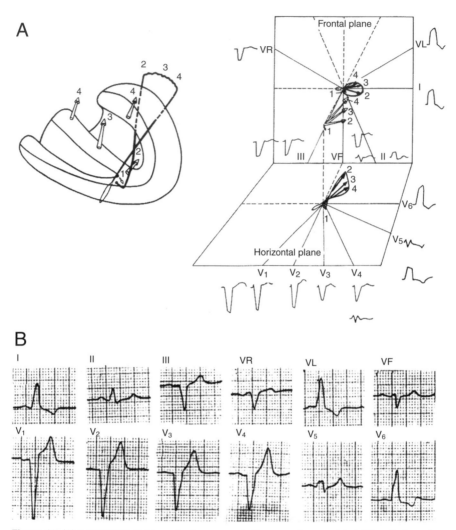

Figure 42 (A) An example of how activation occurs in the case of a complete left bundle branch block and how different lead morphologies are explained by loop–hemifield correlation. (B) A typical ECG in the case of a complete left bundle branch block.

If four intraventricular fascicles are considered to exist, namely, right bundle branch, trunk of the left bundle branch, superoanterior division and inferoposterior division of the left bundle (Figures 5 and 17), besides the isolated blocks of just one fascicle, blocks of two fascicles (bifascicular block) or three fascicles (trifascicular) may exist.

We will now comment on the diagnostic criteria in the different most important types of ventricular blocks.

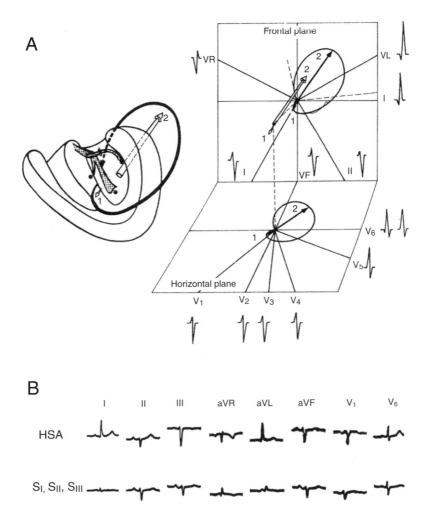

A

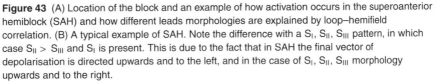

B

| | I | II | III | aVR | aVL | aVF | V₁ | V₆ |

HSA

S_I, S_II, S_III

Figure 43 (A) Location of the block and an example of how activation occurs in the superoanterior hemiblock (SAH) and how different leads morphologies are explained by loop–hemifield correlation. (B) A typical example of SAH. Note the difference with a S_I, S_{II}, S_{III} pattern, in which case $S_{II} > S_{III}$ and S_I is present. This is due to the fact that in SAH the final vector of depolarisation is directed upwards and to the left, and in the case of S_I, S_{II}, S_{III} morphology upwards and to the right.

Complete right bundle branch block (RBBB)
(Table 6 and Figure 40)

This represents a total block of activation of the right ventricle (global block). In this situation, activation of RV is through the septum from the left side and originates the formation of vectors 3 and 4, which explains the global change in the QRS loop. The classical electrocardiographic morphologies, which result

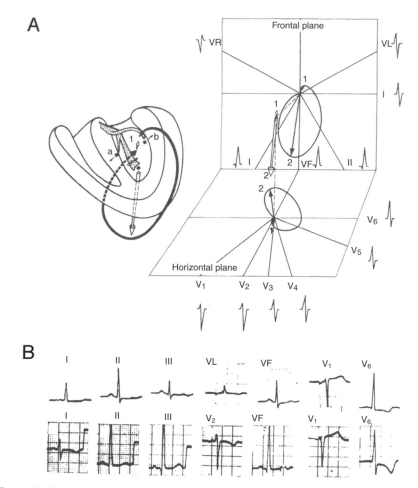

Figure 44 (A) Location of the block and an example how activation occurs in the case of inferoposterior hemiblock (IPH) and how different leads morphologies are explained by loop–hemifield correlation. (B) A patient with ÂQRS around +50° (above) who presented suddenly, without any change in the clinical setting, and ECG showing ÂQRS around +90° (below). This is a typical example of the inferoposterior hemiblock (see the text).

from the loop–hemifield correlation in frontal and horizontal planes, are shown in Figure 40.

Blockade location, both in complete and partial blocks, is usually proximal (see above). Nevertheless, the distal (peripheral) block localization in the distal part of the branch or in the right ventricle Purkinje network is often seen in some congenital heart diseases (Ebstein's disease, post-operative period of Fallot tetralogy, atrial septal defect, etc.) and some cardiomyopathies (arrhythmogenic right ventricular dysplasia), and gives rise to morphologies similar to those of classical complete or partial bundle branch blocks, but in some cases

A   B

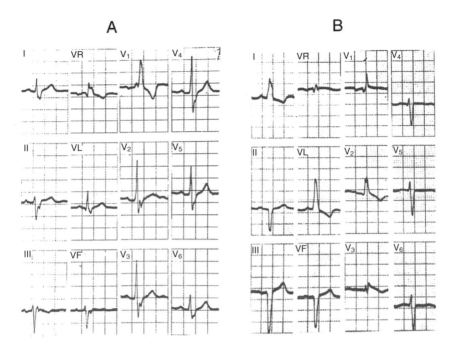

Figure 45 Bifascicular block: (A) complete right bundle branch block + typical superoanterior hemiblock; (B) 'masked' bifascicular block (see the text).

with some specific patterns (Table 4). A tall R wave or an r′SR′ complex in V1, not due to a bundle branch block, can be seen in different situations such as right ventricular enlargement, pre-excitation, lateral infarction and different normal variants (Table 4).

Diagnostic criteria are as follows (Figure 40):
a QRS ≥ 0.12 seconds with mid-final slurrings;
b V1: rsR′ with slurred R wave and a negative T wave;
c V6: qRs with evident S wave slurrings and positive T wave;
d VR: QR with evident R wave slurrings and negative T wave;
e T wave with its polarity opposed to QRS slurrings.
These correspond to type III of the Mexican school (see Table 6).

Partial right bundle branch block (Figure 41)

In this case, activation delay in the entire ventricle is less important. QRS complex duration is less than 0.12 seconds, but V1 still presents rsR′ or rsr′ morphology, but with fewer notches and slurrings. In some cases of right ventricular enlargement, as in an atrial septal defect, due to a delay of activation of some parts of the right ventricle as a consequence of enlargement, a similar pattern may be seen (Figure 32B).

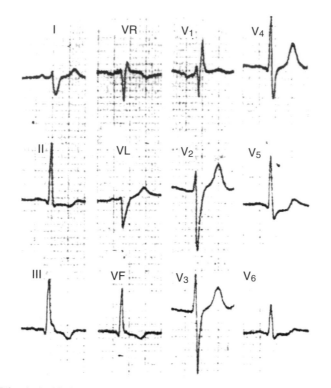

Figure 46 Bifascicular block: complete right bundle branch block + inferoposterior hemiblock in a 56-year-old man with a chronic ischaemic heart disease and without asthenic body-build and right ventricle enlargement (see the text).

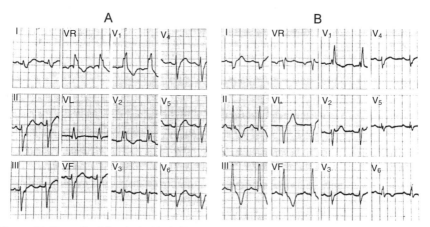

Figure 47 Alternating bifascicular block (Rosenbaum's syndrome). (A) Complete right bundle branch block + superoanterior hemiblock (SAH), and the following day (B) frontal AQRS changed from −60° to +130° as the expression of the appearance of an inferoposterior hemiblock (IPH) instead of SAH.

Table 6 Right ventricular block.

Global: Known as right bundle branch block

1 Third degree (advanced). Morphologies corresponding to type III of the Mexican school [7]: slurred rsR′ in V1 and qRS with slurred S in V6 with QRS ≥ 0.12 s.
2 First degree (partial). Morphologies corresponding to type I: rSr′ in V1 and type II: rSR′ in V1 of the Mexican school with QRS < 0.12 s [7].
3 Second degree. Intermittent block morphology; corresponds to a special type of **ventricular aberrancy**.

Zonal or divisional

Experimentally, it originates ECG morphologies of the S$_I$ S$_{II}$S$_{III}$ or R$_1$ S$_{II}$ S$_{III}$ type [62]. In clinical practice these morphologies are difficult to differentiate from normal variants or RVE (the changes in P and T waves may help). The S$_I$ R$_{II}$ R$_{III}$ morphology must also be explained by inferoposterior hemiblock.

Complete left bundle branch block (LBBB)
(Table 7 and Figure 42)

This represents a total block of the left ventricle activation (global block). In this case, LV activation is through the septum from the right side and differs completely from normal activation. This transseptal activation originates the formation of four vectors characteristic of this type of block and explains the global change in the QRS loop. The classical electrocardiographic morphologies, due to the loop–hemifield correlation in frontal and horizontal planes can be seen in Figure 42.

Distal blocks in the left bundle or in the left ventricle Purkinje network are less frequent than proximal blocks. Distal blocks' morphology is similar to that of classical proximal complete left ventricular blocks, but with more significant final slurrings. Wherever the global block is located (proximal or distal), when

Table 7 Left ventricular block.

Global: Known as left bundle branch block

1 Third degree (advanced). Corresponds to type III of the Mexican school [7]: slurred R in V6 and QS or rS in V1 with QRS ≥ 0.12 s.
2 First degree (partial). Corresponds to types I and II of the Mexican school [7]: isolated R in V6 with more or fewer slurring but QRS < 0.12 s.
3 Second degree. Intermittent block morphology; corresponds to a special type of **ventricular aberrancy**.

Zonal or divisional

• **Hemiblocks** [24]: the block is located in the superoanterior or inferoposterior divisions of the left bundle branch. Superoanterior **hemiblock** originates a qR pattern in lead I and VL and rS in leads II, III, VF while inferoposterior hemiblock originates an RS pattern in lead I and VL and a qR pattern in leads II, III and VF.
• Block of the middle fibres probably produces RS morphologies in V1 [1].

the delay is significant, an R-wave morphology in V6 and a QS complex in V1 with a QRS $\geq$ 0.12 seconds are generated.

   Diagnostic criteria are as follows (Figure 42):

a QRS $\geq$ 0.12 seconds, sometimes over 0.16 seconds, especially with mid-portion slurrings;

b V1: QS or rS with a tiny r wave and positive T wave;

c I and V6: single R with its peak after the initial 0.06 seconds;

d VR: QS with positive T wave;

e T wave with its polarity usually opposed to QRS complex slurrings.

   This corresponds to type III of the Mexican school [7] (see Table 7). In the case of LBBB due to ischaemic cardiomyopathy, we have demonstrated that the voltage of QRS in V3 is smaller than in the case of LBBB due to idiopathic cardiomyopathy.

Partial left bundle branch block

In this case, the entire ventricle activation delay is less significant due to QRS complex duration being less than 0.12 seconds although presents a QS complex or a tiny 'r' wave in V1 and a single R wave in I and V6. This is explained by the fact that the first vector responsible for the formation of 'r' in V1 and q in V6 is not formed because the delay in activation is balanced by the forces of the right ventricle although the rest of the LV activation is normal. Similar morphology due to the presence of septal fibrosis may also participate in the disappearance of 'q' in V6. This pattern is often present in the case of left ventricular enlargement [1,19] (Figures 36 and 37).

Zonal (divisional) left ventricular block

The stimulus is blocked in either the superoanterior or inferoposterior division of the left branch (hemiblocks) (Figures 17D, 43, 44). We will comment only on the electrocardiographic criteria of well-established (complete) superoanterior and inferoposterior hemiblocks.

   According to Rosenbaum and Elizari [24], a change in left intraventricular activation exists in both hemiblocks; as a consequence the blocked area is depolarised with certain delay, which explains the typical electrocardiographic changes that can be seen.

Superoanterior hemiblock (SAH) (Figure 43)

In the upper part of Figure 43, location of the block and activation of the left ventricle in the case of a superoanterior hemiblock and the loop–hemifield correlation in frontal and horizontal planes can be seen. In the lower part, a typical example of a superoanterior hemiblock is shown, as well as differences with the S_I, S_{II}, S_{III} pattern (Figure 43 – see the caption).

Diagnostic criteria are as follows [24]:

a QRS complex duration < 0.12 seconds.

b ÂQRS deviated to the left (mainly between −45° and −75°). Inferior necrosis, type-II Wolff–Parkinson–White (WPW) syndrome and an S_I, S_{II}, S_{III} pattern should all be ruled out (Figure 43, lower part).

c I and VL: qR; in advanced cases with slurrings especially in the descending part of R wave.

d II, III and VF: rS with $S_{III} > S_{II}$ and $R_{II} > R_{III}$.

e An S wave seen up to V6, with intrinsicoid deflection in V6 < VL.

Inferoposterior hemiblock (IPH) (Figure 44)

In order to make this diagnosis, both typical electrocardiographic morphology and clinical conditions, mainly the absence of right ventricular enlargement and asthenic habit have to be present. Usually, it is considered that evidence of left ventricular abnormalities must exist. Location of the block and activation of the left ventricle in the case of an inferoposterior hemiblock, together with the typical electrocardiographic morphology, in frontal and horizontal planes, explained by the loop–hemifield correlation can be seen in Figure 44A. In this case the diagnosis is assured since the ECG pattern appeared abruptly (Figure 44B – see the caption).

Diagnostic criteria are as follows:

a QRS complex duration < 0.12 seconds.

b ÂQRS shifted to the right (between +90° and ≥110° for some authors and +140°).

c I and VL: RS or rS.

d II, III and VF: qR; in advanced cases with slurrings especially in the descending part of R wave.

e Precordial leads: S wave up to V6, with an intrinsicoid deflection time in V6 < VF.

Bifascicular blocks

We will comment on the electrocardiographic criteria of the two most characteristic bifascicular blocks: complete right bundle branch block plus anterosuperior hemiblock and complete right bundle branch block plus inferoposterior hemiblock.

Complete right bundle branch block plus superoanterior hemiblock

Diagnostic criteria are as follows (Figure 45):

a QRS complex duration > 0.12 seconds.

b QRS complex morphology: the first portion is directed like the superoanterior hemiblock, upwards and to the left, while the second portion is directed as in the advanced global right bundle branch block, anteriorly and to the right (Figure 45A). If a significant left delay exists, it can counteract the right forces; this gives rise to anterior but left, final forces, so a tall R wave can be seen in

V1, but without an S wave in I and, occasionally, in V6. In this case, a complete left bundle branch block appears to exist in the frontal plane and a complete right bundle branch block in the horizontal plane ('masked' block) [25] (Figure 45B).

Complete right bundle branch block plus inferoposterior hemiblock
(Figure 46)
Diagnostic criteria are as follows:
a QRS complex duration > 0.12 seconds.
b QRS complex morphology: the first portion of the QRS complex is directed downwards, as in the inferoposterior hemiblock, while the second portion is directed anteriorly and to the right like in the complete right bundle branch block. To make this diagnosis it is necessary that some clinical conditions exist, as in the case of an isolated inferoposterior hemiblock (see above).

Trifascicular blocks

Several possibilities exist. To list them all, even superficially, is beyond the scope of this book [1]. The most frequent cases are as follows: (a) a right bundle branch block alternating with the blockade of one of two left bundle branch divisions (**Rosenbaum's syndrome**) [1] (Figure 47), and (b) bifascicular blocks with a long PR segment. It must be borne in mind that a long PR segment may also be due to a block at a proximal location (His bundle), thus electrophysiologic studies are required to confirm their occurrence. The ECG evidence that block exists in three fascicles even if it is transient means that a complete paroxysmal AV block may suddenly occur and strongly recommends pacemaker implantation.

CHAPTER 10

Ventricular pre-excitation

Ventricular pre-excitation is considered to exist when the electric stimulus reaches the ventricles earlier (early excitation) than normal (via the specific conduction system). Early excitation is explained by the fact that some accelerated conduction pathways connect the atria with the ventricles, the so-called Kent bypass tract (**WPW-type pre-excitation)** [26], or is a consequence of the existence of an atrio-His tract or simply due to the presence of an accelerated AV conduction (**short PR pre-excitation named Lown–Ganong–Levine syndrome**) [27]. The importance of pre-excitation lies in its association with supraventricular tachycardias, its potential danger of triggering malignant arrhythmia, and the risk of its being mistaken (in the case of the WPW preexcitation) for other processes (*vide infra*).

WPW-type pre-excitation

Electrocardiographic diagnosis is made by the presence of a short PR interval plus QRS abnormalities due primarily to the presence of slurrings, in its beginning (delta wave) (Figure 48).

Short PR interval
The PR interval generally lasts between 0.08 and 0.11 seconds. WPW-type pre-excitation can exist with a normal PR interval in the presence of (a) preexcitation via the Mahaim tracts, (b) conduction block in the anomalous pathway, and (c) pre-excitation far from the sinus node (left side), frequently with a long anomalous pathway. Only the comparison with the baseline ECG tracing without pre-excitation will confirm whether the PR interval is shorter than the basal, which may confirm the diagnosis.

Ventriculogram abnormalities [28,29] (Figures 48–50)
QRS complexes show an abnormal morphology with a width greater than that of the baseline QRS complex (often >0.11 seconds) and characteristic initial slurring (delta wave), which are secondary to the initial activation through the contractile myocardium where there are few Purkinje fibres. Different degrees of pre-excitation (of delta wave) may be observed (Figure 48).

QRS complex morphology in different surface ECG leads depends on the location of the epicardial zone of earlier excitation. The vector of the first 20 ms on the ECG (first vector of the delta wave, which can be measured in the ECG) is located at different sites of the frontal plane according to where the earlier ventricular epicardial excitation occurred first (Figure 49). Accordingly, the

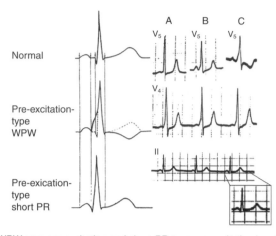

Figure 48 Left: WPW-type pre-excitation and short-PR-type pre-excitation in relation to the normal activation. Right: (top) delta waves of different magnitudes (A) minor pre-excitation; (B and C) significant pre-excitation; (middle) three consecutive QRS with evident pre-excitation; (below) short-PR-type pre-excitation.

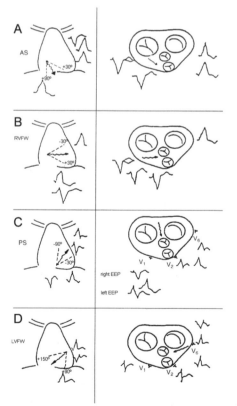

Figure 49 Morphologies in WPW-type pre-excitation according to the ventricular early epicardial pre-excitation (EEP) due to location of the accessory AV pathway in the following zones: (A) right anteroseptal (AS) – orginates EEP directed between +30° and +90°; (B) right ventricular free wall (RVFW) – originate EEP between +30° and −30°; (C) posteroseptal (PS) – originates EEP to the left and above, beyond −30°; and (D) left ventricular free wall (LVFW) originates EEP to the right beyond +90° and below.

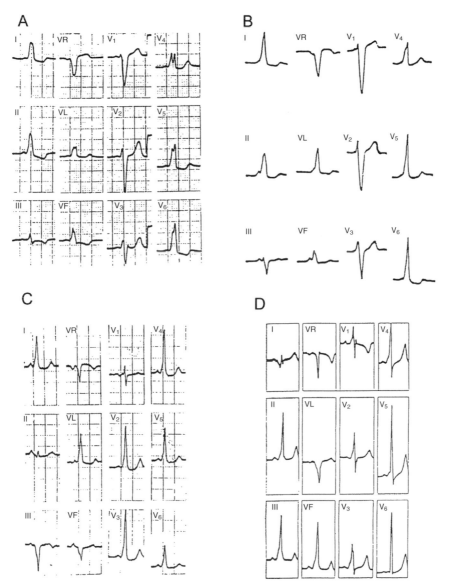

Figure 50 ECG examples in the WPW-type pre-excitation with accessory AV pathway located in the right anteroseptal zone: delta wave $\cong +40°$ (A); right ventricular free wall: delta wave $\cong +10°$ (B); posteroseptal zone: delta wave $\cong -40°$ (C); and left ventricular free wall: delta wave $\cong +120°$ (D).

WPW-type pre-excitation may be divided into four types (Figure 49) [1]. Examples of these four types may be seen in Figure 50.

Different algorithms exist to predict the location of the anomalous pathway [29] (Figure 51). However, electrophysiologic studies are required to assure its exact location. The exact place of the anomalous path is critical for performing its correct ablation, a procedure performed to suppress pre-excitation and

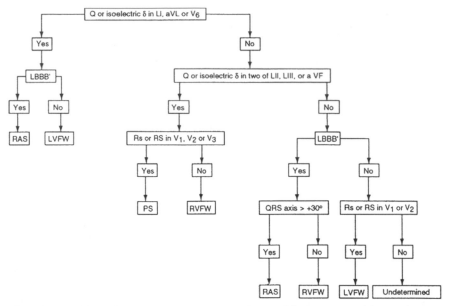

Figure 51 Algorithm to locate the accessory pathway in one of the four zones: right anteroseptal (RAS), right ventricular free wall (RVFW), posteroseptal (PS), and left ventricular free wall (LVFW).

avoid recurrence of supraventricular paroxysmal tachycardias so frequent in these patients.

Repolarisation abnormalities

Repolarisation is altered except in the cases with minor pre-excitation. Its changes are secondary to depolarisation alteration and are more pathologic with its polarity more opposed to that of the R wave when pre-excitation is greater.

Differential diagnosis of Wolff–Parkinson–White-type pre-excitation

Types A and B can be mistaken for a left bundle branch block (Figures 49A, B, 50A and B), type C pre-excitation can be mistaken for an inferolateral infarction, right bundle branch block or right ventricular enlargement (Figures 49C and 50C), and type D can be mistaken for lateral infarction or right ventricular enlargement (Figures 49D and 50D). In all these cases, a short PR interval and the presence of a delta wave are decisive data for the diagnosis of WPW-type pre-excitation.

Spontaneous or provoked changes in anomalous morphology

Changes in the degree of pre-excitation are frequent. Pre-excitation can increase if stimulus conduction through the AV node is depressed (vagal manoeuvres, drugs, etc.) and can decrease if, in contrast, AV node conduction is enhanced (physical exercise, etc.).

Diagnosis by surface ECG of more than one pathway [28]

In sinus rhythm: (a) qrS or qRs pattern in V1; (b) change from one pattern to another.

During tachycardia: (a) wide and narrow QRS alternans; (b) RR alternans; (c) change in P'-wave morphology.

WPW pre-excitation and arrhythmias

Paroxysmal arrhythmias in patients with a WPW electrocardiographic pattern constitute **the WPW syndrome**. Patients with WPW pre-excitation frequently present **macroreentry paroxysmal tachycardia**. Indeed, approximately 40–50% of paroxysmal tachycardias are attributed to a reentry including an accessory pathway. The tachycardia usually starts when a premature atrial beat is blocked in the anomalous pathway that allows reentry by retrograde conduction through the accessory pathway. In this situation, ventricular depolarisation occurs through the normal way, so that during tachycardia the QRS does not show pre-excitation (**orthodromic tachycardia**) (Figure 52). In less than 10% of paroxysmal tachycardia cases, anterograde ventricular depolarisation occurs through the accessory pathway (right-sided slow atriofascicular pathway or classical Mahaim fibres), resulting in a very wide QRS (**antidromic tachycardia**) [1].

Also, atrial fibrillation and flutter episodes are more frequent than in the general population. This is attributed to the rapid retrograde conduction via the abnormal pathway of a ventricular premature complex that may reach the atria during a vulnerable atrial period. Another possibility is that paroxysmal tachycardia triggers other arrhythmias such as atrial fibrillation/flutter. The risk of these arrhythmias is twofold. Firstly, atrial fibrillation/flutter in patients with an ECG pattern of WPW can be mistaken for sustained ventricular tachycardia, with the consequences associated with it (Figure 53). Secondly, in the presence of atrial fibrillation or flutter, the potential danger is that the accessory pathway may transmit to the ventricle more stimuli than normal, facilitating the possibility of reaching the ventricle in its vulnerable period. Consequently, this can result in the triggering of **ventricular fibrillation and sudden death** (Figure 54). This phenomenon explains some sudden death cases, particularly in young individuals. Fortunately, this occurs only very rarely.

Surface ECG criteria that permit the **identification of patients at higher risk of sudden death** include the following [30]:

a A very short RR interval (≤220 ms) during spontaneous or induced atrial fibrillation.

b The existence of two or more different types of supraventricular tachyarrhythmias.

c The presence of an underlying heart disease.

d The existence of permanent pre-excitation during Holter recording, with exercise testing and after the administration of certain drugs.

e The presence of multiple accessory pathways.

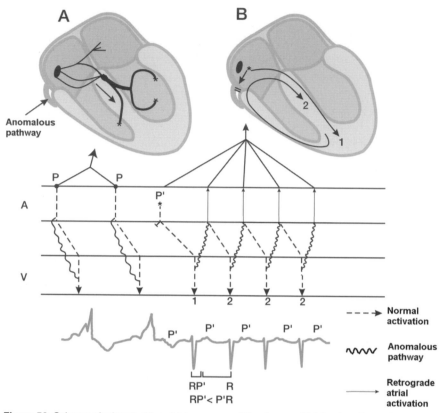

Figure 52 Scheme of a heart with a right accessory AV pathway, which leads to faster than normal AV conduction (short PR) and early activation of part of the ventricles and appearance of abnormal QRS morphology (delta wave) (A). All this may be observed in the first two PQRS complexes of the scheme. The QRS is a summation complex due to initial depolarisation through the accessory AV pathway (curved line) and the rest of depolarisation through the normal AV pathway (discontinuous line). The third P wave is premature (atrial ectopic P′) that finds the accessory AV pathway in the refractory period. Due to this, the impulse is only conducted by normal AV conduction (discontinuous line in AV node) usually with a longer than normal P′R interval, because the AV node is in a relative refractory period. This stimulus originates a normal QRS complex (1) and, due to the fact that the accessory AV pathway is already out of the refractory period, enters it from behind and is conducted retrogradely to the atria generating an evident P′ after the QRS complex (in the case of reciprocal intranodal taquicardia, the P′ is within the QRS complex or can be seen in its final part, modifying the QRS morphology). At the same time, the impulse re-enters and is conducted down to the ventricles via normal AV conduction (B-2). Due to this macroreentry circuit, the reciprocating taquicardia is maintained. The conduction in this circuit is retrograde via accessory AV pathway (curved line) and anterograde via the normal AV conduction (discontinuous line). The RP′ ratio is smaller than the P′R ratio, which is typical of the reciprocating taquicardia that involves an accessory AV pathway.

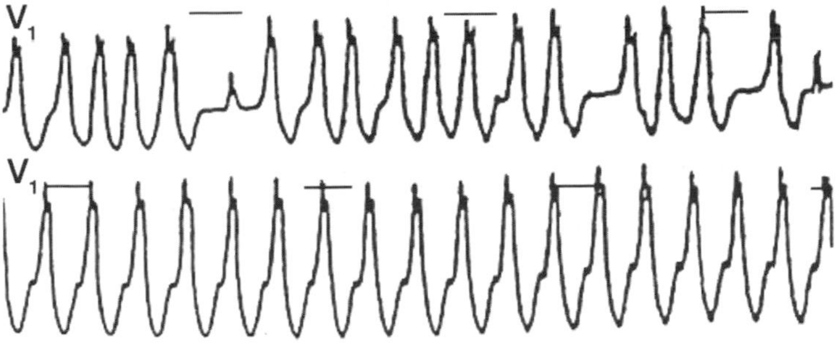

Figure 53 A 50-year-old patient with the Wolff–Parkinson–White syndrome of type IV who presents additionally a crisis of atrial fibrillation (above) and atrial flutter (below) that mimics ventricular taquicardia. The diagnosis of atrial fibrillation is supported by the history taking (to know that the patient presents WPW syndrome) and the following characteristics of the ECG: (1) the wide complexes have very irregular rhythm and are more or less wider (present more or less pre-excitation); (2) the narrow complexes (the fifth and the last one on the top) sometimes are close, last one, and sometimes far, the fifth, to the previous QRS. In the sustained ventricular tachycardia the QRS complexes are regular and in the case of presence of narrow complexes, these are always close to the previous one (capture beats). Below: in the case of WPW syndrome with flutter, the differential diagnosis with sustained ventricular tachycardia based only on ECG is even more difficult.

Short PR type pre-excitation (Lown–Ganong–Levine syndrome) [27] (Figure 48)

This type of pre-excitation described by Lown–Ganong and Levine is evidenced by a short PR interval without changes in QRS morphology [27] (Figure 48). Usually there is not PR segment (Figures 15 and 48). It is impossible to assure with a surface ECG whether it is a pre-excitation occurring via an atrio-His path, which bypasses the AV node slow conduction area and, therefore, does not modify the QRS complex morphology, or it is simply a hyperconductive AV node.

The association with arrhythmias and sudden death is less frequent than in the WPW-type pre-excitation.

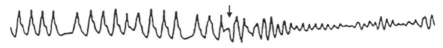

Figure 54 A patient with crisis of atrial fibrillation with a very fast response of the ventricles (> 300 x′) and sometimes very narrow RR intervals (< 200 ms). After a very short RR interval, the crisis of ventricular fibrillation was triggered by a premature ventricular complex (arrow), which had to be resolved by electric cardioversion.

CHAPTER 11

Electrocardiographic pattern of ischaemia, injury and necrosis

Anatomic introduction

The left ventricle has four walls (Figures 55A, B and C). Currently they are named as follows: septal, anterior, lateral and inferior. Classically, the term posterior wall was given to the basal part of the inferior wall that bends upwards [31]. Now the posterior wall is named, according the statement of American Societies of Imaging [32] and the consensus of ISHNE [33], as the inferobasal part of the inferior wall (Figure 55). Conversely, MI of this inferobasal segment (old posterior wall) does not explain the presence of RS in V1, which in turn is due to infarction of the lateral wall [33–35]. The following criteria are crucial to demonstrate it:

a The inferobasal segment depolarises after 40 ms.

b It usually does not bend up.

c The heart is located in an oblique right-to-left position not in a strict posteroanterior position. Therefore, in the case of necrosis of inferobasal segment, the necrosis vector will face V3–V4 instead of V1.

All these arguments are of crucial importance to demonstrate that the MI of the inferobasal segment (old posterior wall) does not explain the presence of RS in V1, which in turn is due to infarction of the lateral wall (see below and Figure 59).

These four walls are divided into 17 segments (Figure 55A–C). Figure 56 represents these segments in the form of a bullseye and the perfusion that the different segments receive from the coronary arteries (B–D). Nevertheless, we should not forget that there exist some variants in coronary flow distribution due to anatomic variants of coronary arteries. In general, in 80% of cases the left anterior descending (LAD) artery is long and wraps the apex, and in around 80% of cases right coronary artery (RCA) dominates left circumflex artery (LCX) (Figure 56A).

As a consequence, the left ventricle may be divided in two zones: **inferolateral** (which encompasses the inferior wall, the inferior part of septal wall, and nearly all lateral wall), perfused by RCA artery and/or LCX and **anteroseptal** (which encompasses the anterior wall, the anterior part of the septal wall and small part of mid-low lateral wall) perfused by the LAD artery (Figure 56A). The lateral wall therefore is perfused especially by LCX and often partly by LAD and RCA. The anteroseptal zone is always perfused by LAD; however, the LAD artery usually also supplies blood to the inferior part of the inferior wall (long LAD that wraps the apex). The RCA perfuses the inferior

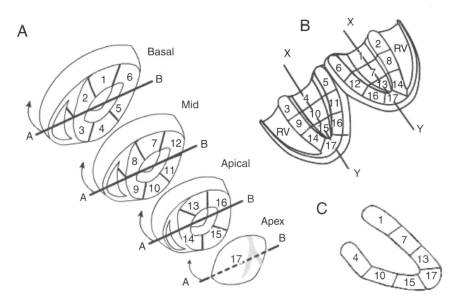

Figure 55 (A) Segments into which the left ventricle is divided, according to the transverse sections (short axis view) performed at basal, medial and apical levels. The basal and medial sections delineate six segments each, while the apical section shows four segments. Together with the apex, they constitute the 17 segments into which the heart can be divided, according to the classification of the American Imaging Societies [32]. Anterior wall corresponds to 1, 7 and 13 segments, inferior wall to 4, 10 and 15 (4 was the old normal posterior wall and now named inferobasal segment), septal to 2, 3, 8, 9 and 14, and lateral to 5, 6, 11, 12 and 16, segment 17 is the apex. (B and C) View of the 17 segments with the heart open on a horizontal longitudinal plane obtained by opening the heart following the line AB of A. and oblique–sagittal (right view) plane obtained following the line XY of B (C).

wall, predominantly the mid-inferior part of the wall and the inferior part of the septum and, in the case of evident RCA dominance, all inferior wall and also part of the lateral wall. The LCX supplies blood to the inferolateral zone, especially the inferobasal part of the inferior wall and the lateral wall by its branch called the oblique marginal (OM) artery. The areas perfused by coronary arteries with the areas of shared perfusion are displayed in Figure 56.

Electrophysiological introduction

Myocardial ischaemia represents a decrease in the perfusion of a certain area of the myocardium **(ischaemic heart disease)** generally due to atherothrombosis. If significant and persistent, it usually leads to tissue necrosis **(myocardial infarction)**. Different degrees or types of clinical ischaemia correspond to different electrocardiographic patterns. The so-called **electrocardiographic pattern of ischaemia is represented by changes in T wave, the ECG pattern of injury by ST changes, while pathologic Q wave classically corresponds to an ECG pattern of necrosis.** In Figure 57, we can observe ionic changes,

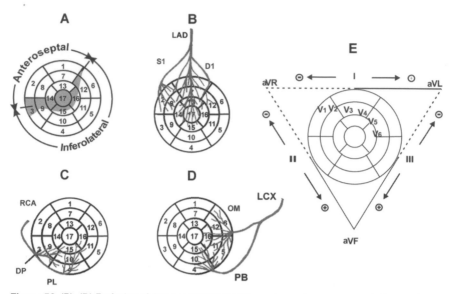

Figure 56 (B)–(D) Perfusion of these segments by the corresponding coronary arteries can be seen in a bullseye perspective. (A) The areas of shared perfusion. (E) The correlation with ECG leads (see the text).

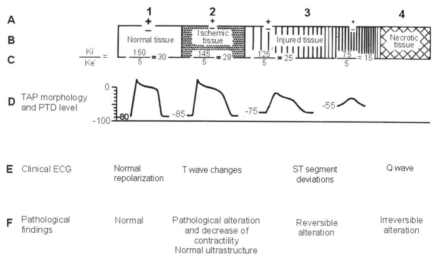

Figure 57 Observe the corresponding electrical charges and ionic changes (A and C), DTP levels and TAP morphologies (D), clinical ECG (E), and pathological finding (F), in different types of tissue (normal, ischaemic, injured and necrotic) (B).

Table 8 Different ECG patterns in acute and chronic ischaemic heart disease and grade of myocardial involvement.

---

1. STE-ACS   First predominant, subendocardial compromise occurs and later, transmural and homogeneous compromise in a heart usually without important previous ischaemia

1.1. Typical patterns

Evolving Q wave MI:

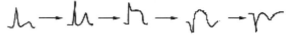

Coronary spasm (atypical STE-ACS):

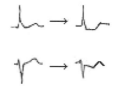

1.2. Atypical patterns (see Figure 72 and Table 11)

2. Non STE-ACS   Compromise sometimes extensive and even transmural, in a heart usually with previous ischaemia

2.1. With evident and predominant subendocardial involvement (see Figure 67A and 68B) and usually increase of LV telediastolic pressure. **"Active ischaemia"**. ST depression that sometimes only appears during pain

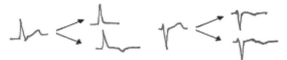

2.2. Without predominant subendocardial involvement. Often represent a post-ischaemic pattern (see p. 74). Flattened or negative T wave may appear (see Figure 60B and 61B and C). Sometimes with negative U wave

3. Chronic heart disease with or without transmural involvement:
—May or may not be present pathological Q wave (see Table 14)
—Also ST deviations and flat/negative T wave may be present
—The presence of "active ischaemia" is only evident if ST/T changes occur during pain or exercise

---

ACS, acute coronary syndrome.

anatomopathologic alterations and electrophysiologic characteristics that accompany different patterns (**ECG pattern of ischaemia, injury and necrosis**). The relationship between the degree of ventricular wall involvement, degree and type of ischaemia and electrocardiographic patterns of ischaemia, injury and necrosis is given in Table 8.

Occlusion of an artery may originate a **direct ECG pattern in leads facing the affected zone** and also **reciprocal (indirect) ECG patterns** (Figures 58 and 59). In **acute coronary syndromes (ACS)** the reciprocal changes ('ups and downs' of

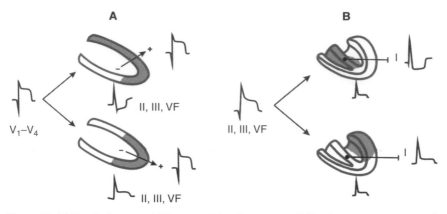

Figure 58 (A) How in the case of ST-segment elevation in precordial leads, as a consequence of LAD occlusion, the ST changes in reciprocal leads (II, III, VF) allow us to identify whether the occlusion is in the proximal (above) or distal LAD (below). (B) How in the case of ST elevation in inferior leads (II, III, VF) the ST changes in other leads, in this case lead I, provide information on whether the inferoposterior infarction is due to RCA (above) or LCX (below) occlusion (see the text).

ST – explained by the ST injury vector theory) (see Figure 58) are important for predicting which is the culprit artery (RCA vs LCX) in the case of ST elevation in II, III, VF (Figure 58A), and where the place of occlusion in LAD in the case of ST elevation in precordial leads (Figure 58B). **Similarly, in the chronic phase** we are able to evaluate tall R and positive T waves in V1–V2 as a mirror image of infarction affecting the lateral wall and not the posterior wall as was thought previously (Figure 59) according to the necrosis vector theory and the correlation with cardiovascular magnetic resonance (CMR) [33–35] (see p. 104).

Henceforth, we will comment on the characteristics of the **ECG pattern of ischaemia, injury and necrosis** observed (see Table 8 and Figure 57) with a gradually decreasing coronary blood flow leading finally to cell death. It must be remembered that a **similar ECG pattern may be observed in various clinical**

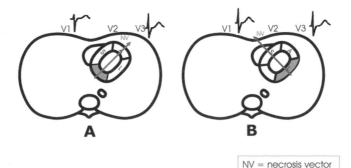

NV = necrosis vector

Figure 59 (A) The correlation with CMR has demonstrated that in the case of infarction of inferobasal segment of the heart (old posterior wall) the infarction vector faces V3 instead of V1, and therefore does not generate RS morphology in V1. On the contrary, (B) in the case of lateral infarction, the infarction vector faces V1 and may generate RS in V1 (see Figures 94 and 95).

situations apart from coronary artery disease. Therefore, in the case of an isolated electrocardiogram with a pattern suggestive of ischaemia, injury or necrosis, it is always mandatory to perform exhaustive differential diagnosis (Tables 9–12 and 16).

Electrocardiographic pattern of ischaemia

The ECG pattern of ischaemia (changes of T wave) is recorded in an area of myocardium in which a delay of repolarisation occurs (Figure 57(2)) as a consequence of decrease in blood perfusion of smaller degree than what is necessary to develop an injury pattern, or the pattern is a consequence of ischaemia but not due to "active ischaemia" (post ischaemic changes).

From the experimental point of view, ischaemia may be subepicardial, subendocardial or transmural. **From the clinical point of view only subendocardial and transmural ischaemia exist and the latter is considered to be equivalent to subepicardial owing to its proximity to the explorer electrode.**

Experimentally, the **ECG pattern of ischaemia** (**changes in T wave**) may be recorded in an area of the left ventricle subendocardium or subepicardium in which, as a consequence of a decrease in blood supply (less than needed to generate the ECG pattern of injury) or for other reasons such as cooling the area, **a delay in repolarisation in the affected zone occurs**. If the **ischaemia** is **subendocardial** a **higher than normal positive T wave** is recorded and in the case of **subepicardial ischaemia** (or in clinical practice transmural due to its proximity to the explorer electrode) a **flattened or negative T wave.**

A vector is originated from the zone that as a consequence of ischaemia is not yet fully repolarised and still presents negative charges, and is directed towards the already repolarised area presenting with positive charges (**vector of ischaemia**). In the case of subendocardial ischaemia the vector of ischaemia moves away from the ischaemic zone with late repolarization and originates a taller than normal T wave (Figure 60A). If the zone with late repolarization is subepicardial (or in clinical practice transmural), the vector of ischaemia will explain flattened or negative T wave (Figure 60B).

The second way to explain the electrocardiographic pattern of ischaemia is based on the fact that the ECG curve is a consequence of the **sum of the TAP of the part of a left ventricle distal to an electrode (subendocardial zone) and the part proximal to electrode (subepicardial zone)**. Figure 61 shows how in the case of delay of TAP formation in the subepicardial zone (C and D) the sum of both TAPs explains the formation of flattened or negative T wave (electrocardiographic pattern of subepicardial ischaemia) and in the case of subendocardial ischaemia the delay of TAP in subendocardium will prolong TAP in this zone and the sum of both TAPs explains why the T wave presents higher voltage (B) (electrocardiographic pattern of subendocardial ischaemia).

The T-wave changes, named ECG patterns of ischaemia, are recorded in the second part of repolarisation usually without any evident involvement of the first part of repolarisation (ST segment). This is due to the fact that this pattern appears as a consequence of lengthening of the TAP without changes in the

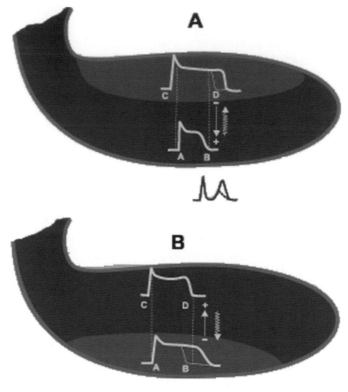

Figure 60 (A) Subendocardial ischaemia. Subepicardial repolarisation is complete, but the TAP in the subendocardium is longer than normal (TAP prolongation further beyond the dotted line) since the subendocardium is not completely repolarised. Thus, the vector head that is generated between the already polarised area in the subepicardium with positive charges and the subendocardial area still with incomplete repolarisation with negative charges due to the ischaemia in that area, named ischaemic vector, is directed from the subendocardium to the subepicardium, even though the direction of the repolarisation phenomenon goes away from it because the direction of the phenomenon (ʌʌ◆) goes from the less ischaemic area to the more ischaemic area. Therefore, the subepicardium faces the vector head (positive charge of the dipole), which explains why the T wave is more positive than normal. In subepicardial ischaemia a similar but inverse phenomenon (B) occurs, which explains the development of flattened or negative T waves.

end of depolarisation and first part of repolarisation (ST segment). As a consequence, usually the T wave of ischaemia follows an isoelectric ST segment.

Alterations of the T wave due to ischaemic heart disease (Table 8)

Negative T wave, known as ECG pattern of subepicardial ischaemia (clinically transmural), secondary to ischaemic heart disease is symmetric and not too wide, with usually an isoelectric ST segment. It is a common finding, especially in a chronic Q-wave-type post-infarction phase, and is a manifestation

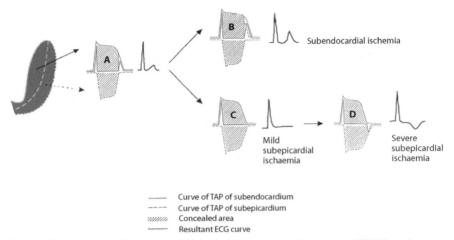

Subendocardial ischemia

Mild subepicardial ischaemia

Severe subepicardial ischaemia

——— Curve of TAP of subendocardium
- - - - Curve of TAP of subepicardium
///////// Concealed area
——— Resultant ECG curve

Figure 61 Explanation of how the sum of the transmembrane action potential (TAP) from the subepicardium and the subendocardium explains the ECG, both in the normal situation (A) , as in the case of subendocardial ischaemia (tall and peaked T wave) (B), and also in mild to severe subepicardial ischaemia (flattened or negative T waves) (C and D). This is due to the fact that the ischaemic area (subendocardium in B and subepicardium in C and D) shows a delay in repolarisation and, consequently, a more prolonged TAP (see the text).

of an ACS, both STE-ACS and non- STE-ACS, (Tables 8 and 11, and Figure 72). In the case of post-myocardial infarction patients, the ECG pattern of ischaemia (negative T wave) is due more to changes of repolarisation induced by Q-wave necrosis than to clinically active ischaemia. In ACS the negative T wave is a consequence of ischaemia but not due to "active" ischaemia. Especially when deep negative T wave is present in VI–V4, it may be the expression of critical LAD occlusion but with still-opened artery or great collateral circulation, (Figure 72C and Table 11A) or it is the expression of reperfusion after fibrinolysisi or PCI. Both cases may evolve to STE-ACS. The presence of negative, usually non-deep, T wave in non-STE-ACS is relatively frequent and probably is not due to "active ischaemia" but is a consequence of it (changes after ischaemia) (Table 11B).

An electrocardiographic pattern of ischaemia is observed in different leads according to an affected zone. **In the case of inferolateral involvement**, T-wave changes are observed in II, III, VF (inferior wall) and/or V1–V2 (mirror image of inferolateral involvement) as positive instead of negative due to the mirror image (Figure 59). In subepicardial inferobasal injury, ST depression will be recorded instead of ST elevation, and in the case of lateral necrosis a tall R wave is recorded instead of Q wave (see below). As we have already commented, we have demonstrated [34,35] that the RS in V1 is due to lateral necrosis and not inferobasal necrosis (Figures 59 and 62). **In anteroseptal involvement**, T-wave changes are found from V1–V2 to V4–V6, and, if mid anterior wall and mid anterior portion of the lateral wall are involved (occlusion proximal to first diagonal), also in V6, I and VL (Figure 63). Also, the involvement of lateral wall areas perfused by LCX may generate not only positive T wave in

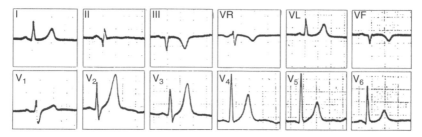

Figure 62 A 55-year-old man with inferolateral infarction according the new classification (Table 15). The T wave in V1–V3, which are tall and peaked, is not the result of anterior subendocardial ischaemia, but of inferolateral subepicardial ischaemia. See also typical Q wave in II–III–AVF and RS in V1 with Rs in V2–V3 seen in this type of infarction (see Figure 58).

V1–V2, but also negative T wave in leads V6, I, VL, and in the chronic phase of infarction, the RS pattern in V1–V2, and/or a "qr" or low "r" may be seen in I, VL, V5–V6, but "QS" in VL. This morphology (QS in VL without Q in V5–V6) is recorded in the case of isolated infarction of the mid anterior wall and mid lateral wall that is due to the first diagonal (D1) occlusion (Figure 64). This pattern is never seen in the case of necrosis of a high lateral wall that is perfused by LCX.

In contrast, the T wave of subendocardial ischaemia is generated during the early phase of ischaemia when predominantly the subendocardial area is involved (Table 8(1)). It is difficult to diagnose owing to its transient characteristics and the difficulties in distinguishing from a normal positive T wave. Therefore requential changes should be evaluated (Figure 65). It is observed in the initial phase of Prinzmetal's angina crisis (coronary spasm) (Table 8(1) and Figure 65) and occasionally in the hyperacute phase of ACS (Figure 72B).

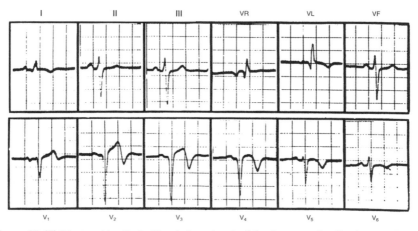

Figure 63 (A) 60-year-old patient with anterior extensive infarction according the new classification (Table 15). Observe in the frontal plane lateral subepicardial ischaemia (negative T waves in I and VL) with a mirror image in II, III, VF and in the HP, the anterolateral subepicardial ischaemia (negative T waves from V1 to V6 and ± V1–V2, and Q waves from V1 to V4 and VL) and low voltage of R in V5–V6 and I.

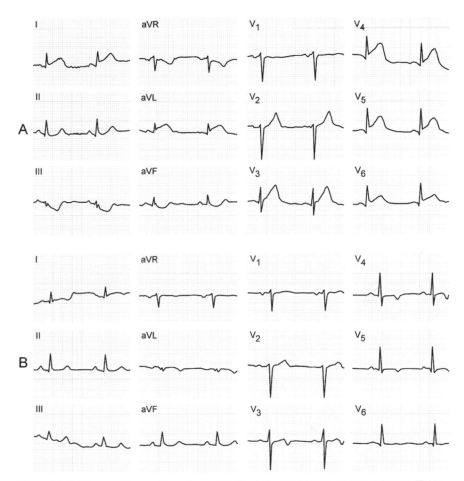

Figure 64 A 67-year-old man with mid-anterior infarction according the new classification (Table 15). (A) Acute phase ST elevation in I, VL and some precordial leads and ST depression in II, III, VF (III > II). (B) Chronic phase: small 'qs' pattern in VL without abnormal Q wave in V5–V6.

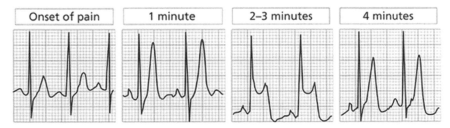

Figure 65 Patient with Prinzmetal's angina crisis. From left to right: four sequences recorded during a crisis of 4-minutes with the Holter recording. Observe how the T wave becomes peaked (subendocardial ischaemia), with a subepicardial injury morphology appearing later, and at the end of the crisis, presenting again a subendocardial ischaemia morphology before the basal ECG returns.

Table 9 Causes of a more positive than normal T wave (apart from ischaemic heart disease) (see Figure 66).

1 Normal variant: vagotonia, sportsmen, the elderly, etc.
2 Acute pericarditis
3 Alcoholism
4 Hyperkalaemia
5 Moderate left ventricular hypertrophy in heart diseases with diastolic overload (e.g. aortic regurgitation)
6 Stroke
7 In advanced AV block (tall and peaked T wave in the narrow QRS complex escape rhythm)
8 In V1–V2 as a 'mirror' image of inferolateral subepicardial ischaemia or secondary to left ventricular hypertrophy

Alterations in T wave in various conditions other than ischaemic heart disease

The most frequent causes, apart from ischaemic heart disease of a negative, flattened or more-positive-than-normal T wave, are summarised in Tables 9 and 10. **Pericarditis is a very important differential diagnosis of the pattern of subepicardial ischaemia**. Apart from clinical characteristics of precordial pain, the ECG in pericarditis shows a pattern of more extensive subepicardial ischaemia with less frequent mirror patterns in the frontal plane, and generally the negativity of T wave is smaller. The examples of different T-wave abnormalities not due to ischaemic heart disease may be observed in Figure 66.

Table 10 Causes of negative or flattened T waves (apart from ischaemic heart disease) (see Figure 60).

1 **Normal variants.** Children, Black people, hyperventilation and women (right precordial leads, etc.); may sometimes be diffuse (global T-wave inversion of an unknown origin). Frequently occurs in women.
2 **Pericarditis.** In this condition, the image is usually extensive, but generally with not such significant negativity.
3 **Cor pulmonale and pulmonary embolism.**
4 **Myocarditis and cardiomyopathies.**
5 **Mitral valve prolapse.** Not always; if it appears, it does so particularly in II, III and VF and/or V5 and V6.
6 **Alcoholism.**
7 **Strokes.** Relatively infrequent.
8 **Myxoedema.** Usually flat T wave or only slightly negative.
9 **Sportsmen.** With or without ST-segment elevation. Hypertrophic cardiomyopathy, especially apical type, must be ruled out.
10 After the **administration of certain drugs** (prenylamine, amiodarone) (flattened T wave).
11 In **hypokalaemia** the T wave can flatten.
12 **Post-tachycardia.**
13 **Abnormalities** secondary to left ventricular hypertrophy or to left bundle branch block.
14 **Intermittent left bundle branch block** and other situations of intermittent abnormal activation (pacemakers, Wolff–Parkinson–White syndrome) 'electrical memory'.

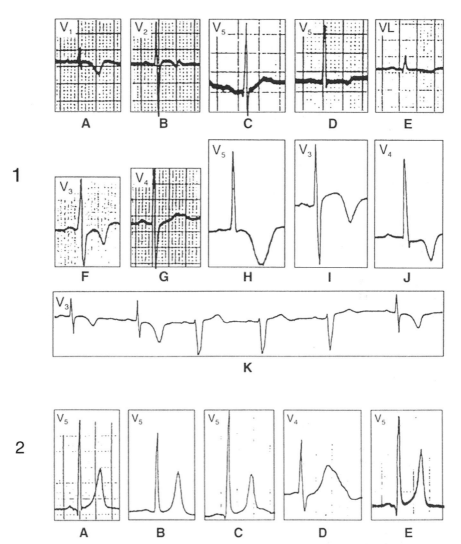

Figure 66 T-wave morphologies in conditions other than from ischaemic heart disease. (1) Some morphologies of flattened or negative T wave: (A and B) V1 and V2 of a healthy 1-year-old girl; (C and D) alcoholic cardiomyopathy; (E) myxoedema; (F) negative T wave after paroxysmal tachycardia in a patient with initial phase of cardiomyopathy; (G) bimodal T with long QT frequently seen after long-term amiodarone administration; (H) negative T wave with a very wide base, sometimes observed in stroke; (I) negative T wave preceded by ST elevation in an apparently healthy tennis player; (J) very negative T wave in the case of apical cardiomyopathy; (K) negative T wave in the case of intermittent LBBB in a patient with no apparent heart disease. (2) Tall peaked T wave in the case of (A) variant of normality (vagotonia with early repolarisation), (B) alcoholism, (C) left ventricular enlargement, (D) stroke and (E) hyperkalemia.

Electrocardiographic pattern of injury

The pattern of injury (changes in ST) is recorded in an area of the myocardium in which an evident **diastolic depolarisation** occurs as a consequence of a significant decrease in blood supply (clinically "active" ischaemia
more significant than that needed to generate the electrocardiographic pattern of ischaemia) (Figure 57(3)). **If the diastolic depolarisation is transmural
its electrocardiographic expression, due to the proximity of the electrodes
to the subepicardium, is subepicardial injury.** The zone with diastolic depolarisation according to the membrane response curve forms a transmembrane action potential with slow ascent and lower area (so-called low-quality
TAP). The changes originated by this diastolic depolarisation in the baseline
(TQ space) are compensated by automatic AC couplet amplifiers in ECG devices and are recorded, due to the presence of 'low-quality' in some TAP,
as changes in ST segment ('ups and downs' of ST). If the ischaemia is very
severe and acute, changes will also affect the last part of QRS. In the leads
facing the injured zone, if the current of injury predominates in the subendocardium ST-segment depression will be recorded and if in the subepicardium (clinically transmural) an ST-segment elevation will be observed.
Mirror patterns also exist, for example, if the subepicardial injury exist in the
lateral-inferobasal wall, ST-segment elevation will be observed in the leads
on the back while ST-segment depression will be seen in V1–V3 as a mirror
image.

   The **ST-segment changes may be explained by two theories**: **vector of injury** or as a consequence of the **sum of TAPs of the two parts of the left ventricle subendocardium plus subepicardium**. According to the theory of **vector of injury**, in the case of injury predominantly in the subendocardial zone
at the end of depolarisation (beginning of systole) the injured zone presents
less negative charges (Figure 67A) and, consequently, a current flow exists
from the zone with more negative charges (less injured zone) to less negative charges (more injured zone). This originates an **injury vector**. This vector
has relatively positive charges (less negative) in the head. Therefore, in cases
of subendocardial injury, both in experimental (Figure 67A(1)) and clinical
state (Figure 67A(2)), in which case the injury is not exclusively but predominantly in the subendocardium, a depression of ST will be recorded. In the
case of subepicardial experimental injury (Figure 67B(1)) and clinically transmural injury (Figure 61B(2)) an ST elevation will be seen (see the caption).
Figure 68 explains how **the theory of the sum of the TAP of subendocardium
and subepicardium** may explain the presence of ST-segment depression in
subendocardial injury or ST-segment elevation in the case of subepicardial
(clinically transmural) injury (see the caption).

   Figure 69 shows different morphologies of subepicardial injury during the
evolution of acute Q-wave anterior myocardial infarction. Figure 70 shows
subendocardial injury pattern observed in course of an acute non-Q-wave
myocardial infarction.

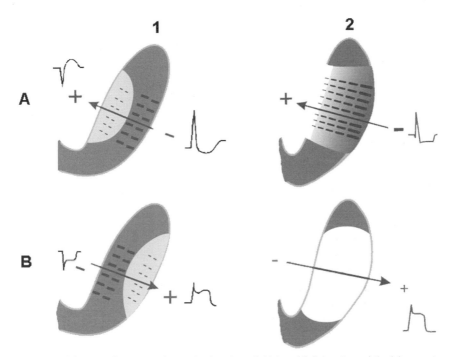

Figure 67 (A) In significant experimental subendocardial injury (1) (injured zone) the injury vector is directed from the non-injured zone (with more negative electric charges) towards the injured zone (with fewer electric charges). The injury vector faces the injured zone, while the ischaemia and necrosis vectors are directed away from the involved area. Therefore, when experimental significant ischaemia (injury) is located in the subendocardium (A-1), the vector is directed from the subepicardium to the subendocardium and generates ST-segment depression in the ECG leads opposing the mentioned zone. In clinical subendocardial injury this is predominantly but not exclusively subendocardial (A-2). (B) In the case of significant experimental subepicardial ischaemia (injured zone), (B-1) the injury vector is directed towards the subepicardium because, in this case, the current flow runs from the subendocardium to subepicardium and generates ST-segment elevation in the precordial ECG leads opposing the mentioned zone. In clinical practice, exclusive subepicardial ischaemia does not exist. The ischaemia that at first is subendocardial, soon becomes transmural. In this case, the surface ECG records the pattern as if it is only subepicardial, due to proximity of the recording electrode to the subepicardium.

Acute coronary syndromes: value of electrocardiographic pattern in classification of acute coronary syndromes, artery occlusion location and risk stratification [36–42]

In around 10–20% of cases of ACS there are confounding factors (left ventricle hypertrophy, bundle-branch block, pacemaker, WPW) that make it more difficult to ascertain the primary change of repolarization induced by ischaemia in ACS [39, 57].

Acute coronary syndromes (ACS) with narrow QRS and without confounding factors, may be classified into two types according to their electrocardiographic expression: with ST-segment elevation (STE-ACS) or without

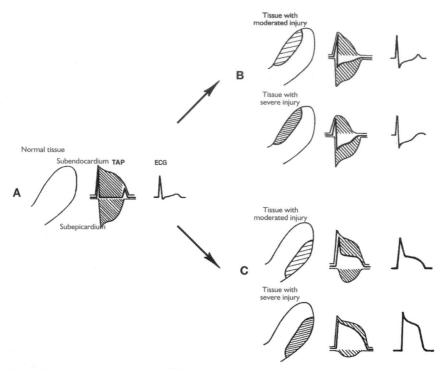

Figure 68 Both the subendocardial (ST depression) and the subepicardial injury (ST elevation) pattern may be explained by the sum of the subendocardial and subepicardial TAPs. The injured zone, subendocardium in (B) and subepicardium in (C), due to the presence of diastolic depolarisation produces a TAP that is slow rising and of less area ('low-quality TAP'). This explains the ECG morphology; ST elevation in subepicardial injury (C) and ST depression in subendocardial injury (B). Clinically, in the case of subepicardial injury pattern the injured zone is transmural but an ST elevation is recorded because the exploring electrode is close to the subepicardium.

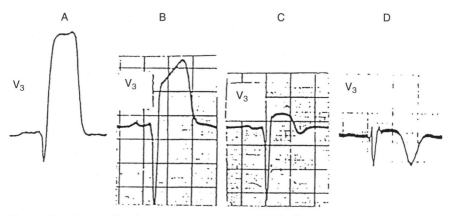

Figure 69 A 72-year-old patient with an extensive anterior infarction. Note the evolutionary patterns: (A) 30 minutes after the onset of pain; (B) 3 hours later; (C) 3 days later; (D) 3 weeks later.

A   B   C   D

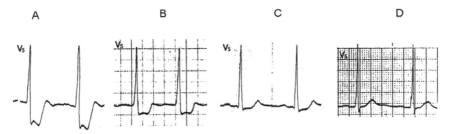

Figure 70 A 65-year-old patient with non-Q-wave infarction. Note the evolutionary patterns from (A) to (D) during the first week until the normalisation of the ST segment.

ST-segment elevation (NSTE-ACS). This classification has a clear clinical significance as the former are treated with fibrinolysis and the latter are not. Figure 71 shows the ECG presentation in ACS and its evolution. Table 11 shows the different ECG patterns seen in the two types of ACS (see below). Very often both ST depression and ST elevation coincide with or without changes of T wave. However, we consider patterns of STE-ACS where the morphology of ST elevation is the predominant and patterns of non STE-ACS where the predominant is the morphology of ST depression. However, the STE-ACS may present some atypical patterns (see Figure 72), and in non STE-ACS include cases of ST segment depression and flat or negative T wave, and even of normal ECG. As a matter of fact, 10–15% of ACS present a normal ECG pattern without pain and even in rare cases the ECG remains normal or nearly normal during the evolution of STE-ACS (grade 1 of ischaemia, p. 92). Sometimes the very subtle ECG changes are transient and appear in the hyperacute phase (pseudonormal ECG pattern) (see Figure 72B).

Acute coronary syndrome with ST-segment elevation: ST-segment elevation acute coronary syndrome (STE-ACS)

Sometimes a small ST-segment elevation but with a convex slope to the isoelectric line may be seen as a normal variant in V1–V2 (Figure 22B). **However, new occurrence of ST elevation over 2 mm in V1–V3 leads and over 1 mm in other leads is considered abnormal and evidence of acute coronary ischaemia in the clinical setting of ACS.** There are the cases of STE-ACS which, thanks to modern treatment, do not lead to Q-wave infarction (in which case we speak about non-Q-wave infarction) and even may not provoke an increase in enzymes and result in aborted infarcts* (unstable angina). Nevertheless, the majority of them will develop a myocardial infarction, usually of Q-wave type (Figure 71).

---

*Due to that we prefer to speak of STE-ACS than STEMI (myocardial infarction). However, both terms may be used independently.

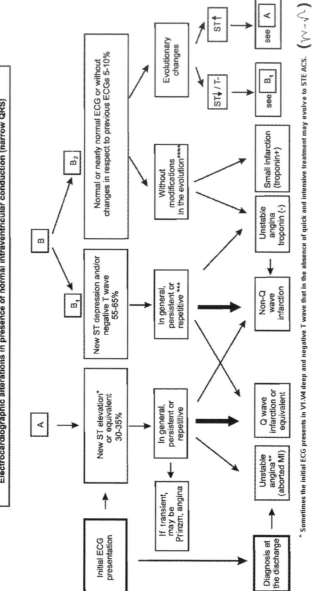

Figure 71 Electrocardiographic alterations observed in patients with acute coronary syndromes presenting with narrow QRS. Observe the initial ECG presentation: (A) ACS with new ST elevation, (B) ACS without new ST elevation with its approximate incidence and final discharge diagnosis according to the evolution.

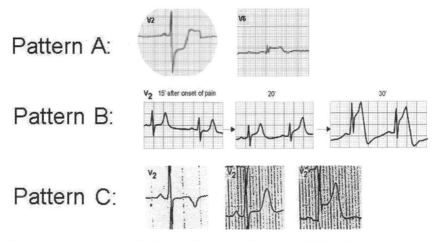

Figure 72 Atypical patterns of ACS with ST elevation. (See text and Table 11.)

ECG patterns seen in STE-ACS
Obviously the typical ECG pattern is the presence of **ST elevation in some leads that predominate over the ST depression usually seen in other leads**. However, the following atypical ECG patterns may be seen in the course of the clinical syndrome of STE-ACS and in its presence the patients have to be considered as STE-MI (Figure 72).
1 Presence of ST depression in V1–V3 more evident than ST elevation in II, III, VF and/or V5–V6, that is usually present in at least some leads. This is a clear case of STE-ACS equivalent due to the presence of injury in the lateral-inferobasal zone that is expressed in V1–V2 as a mirror image – pattern A – (Figure 72A) and we must treat as an STE-ACS (STE-ACS equivalent).
2 In the hyperacute phase of STE-ACS only the pattern of tall positive T wave in V1–V2 due to predominant subendocardial ischaemia, usually preceded by rectified or even mildly negative ST depression, may be seen. This evolving pattern towards STE-ACS may be also considered a STE-ACS pattern – pattern B – (Figure 72B). When the grade of ischaemia is mild a similar pattern of tall and usually wide T wave may remain during the evolution of ACS (Grade 1 of ischaemia, see p. 92).
3 Finally, when **an STE-ACS presents spontaneous or therapeutic reperfusion,** the artery, in case of LAD occlusion, present **a negative and deep T wave in V1 to V4–V5**. In the case that this pattern appears after thrombolysis or PCI, and in the absence of clinical symptoms, this represents a good prognostic sign of reperfusion, and opened artery. However, sometimes it may evolve again to ST elevation if there is an intra-stent thrombosis (dynamic STE-ACS) – pattern C – (Figure 72C). If this pattern appears without a reperfusion treatment it means that the artery is opened, usually partially, or if is completely closed there is great collateral circulation (Wellens sign) [37]. In these cases, it

is necessary to perform coronary angiography as soon as possible, but in the absence of pain not necessarily as an emergency, to check the importance of the occlusion that usually is critical and at proximal level.

Clinical interpretation of ST-segment deviations: prognostic implications
The deviations of ST segment have a great relevance for location of occlusion and for risk stratification and quantification of the myocardial area at risk. We will discuss the following: (A) the importance of deviations of ST segment for location of area at risk; (B) the usefulness of the sum of ST deviations for the quantification of ischaemia; and (C) the ST morphology to detect the grade of ischaemia.

A) Location of occlusion and area at risk

ST-segment elevation is seen predominantly in precordial leads in the case of LAD occlusion and in inferior leads in the case of RCA or LCX occlusion.

Proximal LAD occlusion (before D1 and S1 arteries) as well as occlusion of dominant RCA proximal to right ventricle branches or rarely proximal occlusion of very dominant LCX have the worst prognosis. Therefore, to predict with high accuracy a site of occlusion in an early phase of SCA has therapeutical repercussion in helping us to make decisions regarding the need for urgent reperfusion strategies (PCI, surgery). Careful analysis of ST-segment deviations ('ups and downs') in the ECG recorded at admission may predict the culprit artery and occlusion location. Such a diagnostic approach is based on the **concept of injury vector**. We should remember that ST-segment elevation is found in leads that face the head of an injury vector, while in the opposed leads ST-segment depression can be recorded as a mirror pattern since these leads face the tail of an injury vector (Figure 58).

Figure 73 shows in detail **the algorithm that allows us to predict the site of LAD occlusion in the case of ACS with ST-segment elevation in precordial leads, and Figure 74 the shows the algorithm to follow in the case of ACS with ST-segment elevation in inferior leads, which allows us to distinguish between RCA and LCX occlusion** [39,40], and in the case of RCA occlusion. Later on we have to look for the ECG criteria to know if the occlusion is proximal or distal (Figure 75) [41]. Let us comment in detail on these two algorithms.

1. Dominant ST-segment elevation in precordial leads [39]. This pattern indicates evolving MI of the anteroseptal zone due to an **occlusion in the LAD (Figure 73 and Table 11)**. The only exception is in rare cases with occlusion of a very dominant RCA proximal to right ventricle marginal branches that may present ST elevation in V1 to V3–V4, sometimes greater than ST elevation in inferior leads but usually with the ST elevation in V1 greater than in V3–V4. The cases of distal occlusion of LAD may also present ST elevation in anterior and inferior leads but usually with the ST elevation in V1 less than in V3 [42]. The inferoapical zone is often involved in the case of a long LAD that wraps the apex (occurring in >80% of cases).

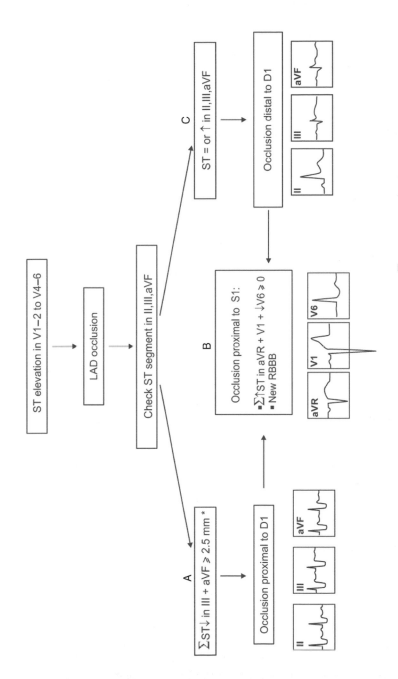

* cases with ST depression < 2.5 mm are difficult to classify in respect to D1, but if $\sum\uparrow$ST aVR + V1 + $\downarrow$ ST V6 < 0, are usually distal to S1.

Figure 73 Algorithm to precisely locate the LAD occlusion in the case of an evolving myocardial infarction with ST elevation in precordial leads (see the text for details).

Table 11 ECG patterns of ACS seen in emergency services at admission.

A   ECG patterns in STE-ACS as the most predominant pattern
1   **Typical:** ST elevation in frontal or horizontal planes with mirror image of ST depression in other leads

2   **Atypical:**
Equivalent: ST depression in V1–V3 obten with smaller ST elevation in II, III, VF/V5–V6 (pattern A, Figure 72) or even without ST elevation in these leads. Often ST elevation in posterior (back) leads

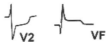

Patterns without ST elevation during some period of the evolving process
   • **Hyperacute phase.** Tall T wave with rectified or even small ST depression (pattern A, Figure 72)

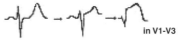

   • **Deep negative T wave in V1 to V4-5.** May be seen as expression of critical LAD occlusion but without necrosis or after fibrinolysis or PCI (**reperfusion pattern**). In both cases may evolve to an STE-ACS (pattern C, Figure 72)

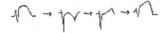

B   ECG patterns in Non-STE-ACS
1   **ST depression as the most predominant pattern**
In ≥ 7 leads (circumferential involvement) with ST elevation in VR
Corresponds to 3-vessel disease or critical LMT subocclusion or equivalent (LAD + CX). If T wave is negative in V4–V6 usually is LMT

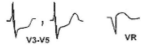

In less than 7 leads (regional involvement) with ST elevation in VR
May be 2–3 vessel disease but with one culprit artery. more frequently in leads with dominant R wave. Cases of worst prognosis present ST depression in V4–V6 and in FP, with negative T wave

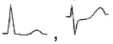

2   **Flat or negative T wave as the most predominant pattern**
The negativity of T wave usually < 2–3 mm. Sometimes a negative U wave may be seen

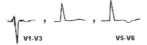

3   **Normal ECG, nearly normal or unchanged during ACS**

C   ECG patterns in presence of confounding factors, LVH, LBBB, PM, WPW

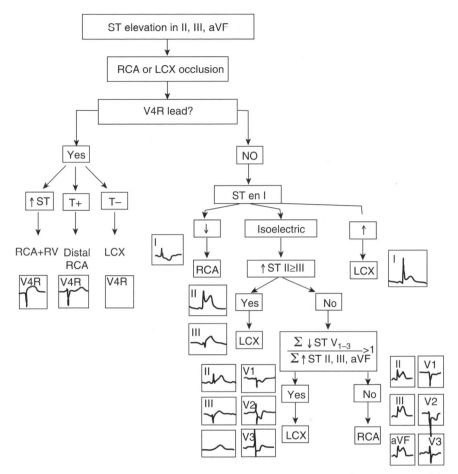

Figure 74 Algorithm to predict the culprit artery (RCA vs LCX) in the case of evolving myocardial infarction with ST elevation in inferior leads (see the text for details).

The occlusion may be proximal to the first septal artery (S1) and first diagonal (D1) (20–45%), between S1 and D1 (30%) or distal to S1 and D1 (10–30%). A sequential approach to ECG analysis based on 'ups and downs' of the ST segment allows us to predict the site of LAD occlusion with high accuracy. The most important ECG changes permitting prediction of proximal or distal occlusion of LAD can be found in inferior leads. Let us comment on the algorithm of Figure 73.

(a) The sum of ST depression in leads III plus VF ≥ 2.5 mm suggests LAD occlusion proximal to D1 (Figure 73A). This is the mirror image of ST elevation in VL. However, in our experience, the sum of ST depression in III + VF ≤ 2.5 mm is a more specific sign than the presence of ST elevation in

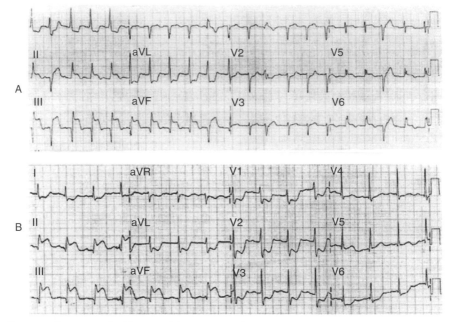

Figure 75 Two cases of ACS due to RCA occlusion: (A) at proximal and (B) at distal level.

VL >1 mm. The affected myocardium is very large and involves a great part of the anteroseptal zone of the heart. Therefore, the injury vector points not only to the front but also upwards because the area of injured myocardium of the anteroseptal zone is much greater than the injured myocardium of the inferolateral zone (even in the case of long LAD) and is consequently recorded as ST elevation in precordial leads and VL and ST depression in inferior leads (Figure 58A). Cases that are difficult to classify are those that present ST depression in III + VF < 2.5 mm. In our experience this sign is more specific for proximal LAD occlusion than the presence of ST elevation in VL > 1 mm.

(b) If ST-segment depression in III and aVF is accompanied by ST elevation in VR and/or V1 and/or by ST depression in V6, occlusion of LAD is more probably proximal not only to D1 but also to S1 (high proximal occlusion) (Figure 73B) since the head of the injury vector also faces the VR and V1 leads and V6 faces the tail of the injury vector. **When ST depression in II, III, VF ≥ 2.5 mm is not accompanied by ST depression in V6 and/or elevation of ST in VR or V1, the occlusion is between S1 and D1.**

(c) Isoelectric or elevated ST segment in II, III, and VF leads suggests LAD occlusion distal to D1 (Figure 73C). In these cases, the affected anteroseptal zone is not very large and if LAD wraps the apex, the injured part of the inferior wall may be equal to or even more significant than the injured anterior wall. In this case, the injury vector points to the front but also a little below (Figure 58A).

2. Dominant ST-segment elevation in inferior leads [40]. This pattern indicates evolving MI of the inferolateral zone due to **occlusion RCA (≅80% of cases) or LCX (≅20% of cases)**. Usually, patients with MI due to RCA occlusion have worse prognosis than those with occluded LCX artery mainly due to the cases with concomitant right ventricle involvement, although the prognosis is also bad in rare cases of proximal occlusion of very dominant LCX. The following sequential algorithm (Figure 74) allows predicting the culprit artery (RCA or LCX) in the case of an evolving MI of the inferolateral zone. The sequential approach that we have to adopt is as follows.

(a) First, right precordial leads should be checked [37]. If these leads are recorded, the morphology of ST/T may identify the place of occlusion (Figure 74). As the changes in right precordial leads are transient, and in clinical practice right precordial leads are often not recorded, we may look for criteria in 12-lead ECG.

(b) We should start by checking how is the ST segment in lead I: an ST-segment depression in lead I points to RCA as the culprit artery (>95% of cases) (the injury vector is directed not only downwards, ST-segment elevation in II, III, VF, but also to the right, generating ST-segment depression in lead I). ST-segment elevation in **lead I indicates that LCX is the affected artery** because the injury vector is directed not only downwards but also to the left (Figures 58B and 74). Only in the case of extremely dominant RCA or LCX have we found that this rule may fail.

In **the case of isoelectric ST** in lead I both RCA and LCX may be a culprit artery. Thus, **we must check whether ST elevation in lead II is equal or greater than ST elevation in lead III. In this case, the affected artery is usually LCX** (the injured vector is directed downwards and leftwards) (Figure 73C). **If it is the contrary (ST elevation III>II), although RCA is the most probable culprit artery, some doubts may exist.**

To be sure, we have to proceed to the **third step: to check the ratio of the sum of ST-segment depression in V1–V3 divided by the sum of ST-segment elevation in II, III, VF. If this ratio is over 1, the affected artery is LCX, if it is equal to or less than 1, RCA is the culprit artery** (Figure 74).

(c) Once we have determined by ECG (Figure 74) with high probability that RCA is the culprit artery, **we may use other ECG criteria to predict proximal versus distal occlusion of RCA** [41]. The right ventricle involvement that usually accompanies proximal RCA occlusion may be determined on the basis of ST changes in right precordial leads (V3R, V4R) [37] (see Figure 74). Nevertheless, ST changes in these leads, though very specific, disappear in the early stage of the evolution of MI. As already stated, another important disadvantage of the diagnosis based on these leads is that they are often not recorded in Emergency Rooms. Thus, the real value of these changes is limited. Therefore, other criteria based on ST changes in lateral or precordial leads have been used to predict the site of RCA occlusion. **In our experience, the**

criterion of isoelectric or elevated ST in V1 has the highest accuracy in predicting proximal RCA occlusion [41] (Figure 75). We have to remember that in these cases the ST elevation in V1 may last till V3 but with V1/V3 ratio over 1 [42].

B) Quantification of the ischaemia

The sum of ST changes in different leads is an easy way to help estimate the myocardium at risk (>15 mm usually represent important area at risk) [36]. However, there are some limitations. In case of STE-ACS due to very proximal RCA occlusion before the artery of the right ventricle, the ST depression in V1–V2 is frequently isodiphasic (without ST deviations). Meanwhile, in many cases of small MI due to distal RCA occlusion, there is an ST depression in these leads.

C) Grade of ischaemia

The morphology of QRS-ST may suggest the intensity of ischaemia: according to Birnbaum–Sclarovsky [38], the patients with STE-ACS that 'sweeps upwards' the QRS and presents a ratio J point/R wave >0.5 has a Grade 3 ischaemia (Figure 72B). The patients with tall permanent T wave have the lowest degree of ischaemia (Grade 1), and finally the patients with ST elevation without QRS distortion have ischaemia Grade 2.

> To sum up, in patients with an ACS with ST elevation, the 12-lead surface ECG recorded at admission may give us a presumptive diagnosis of a culprit artery, site of the occlusion and area at risk, and quantification and grade of ischaemia [37,38]. (See Figures 73 and 74.)

Acute coronary syndromes without ST-segment elevation [43,44]

This group includes the cases of ACS that present with new ST depression and/or new flattened or negative T wave (including negative U waves) in two or more consecutive leads as the most prominent ECG changes (Table 11B), after the exclusion of all atypical cases of STE-ACS (Table 11A). The ST segment depression change ≥0.5 mm occurring in two consecutive leads is already considered sufficient for the diagnosis (Figure 79), although the prognosis is worst when there are more leads involved and the ST depression is more evident. Cases of ACS with normal ECG analysis included.

Non STE-ACS with **ST depression in 7 or more leads (circumferential involvement)** have the worst prognosis as they usually correspond to a left main trunk (LMT) subocclusion and/or three vessel disease occlusion. Negative T wave in V4–V6 is often present in case of LMT involvement. In these cases, generally ST elevation in VR as a mirror image can be observed [43] (Figures 76 and 77).

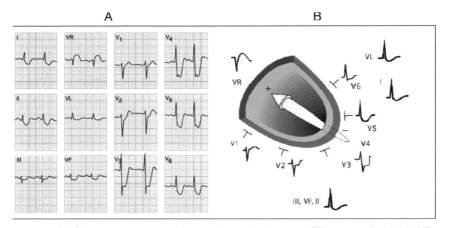

Figure 76 (A) ST-segment depression in more than eight leads and ST-segment elevation in VR in the case of ACS due to the involvement of the left main coronary artery. Note that the maximum depression occurs in V3–V4 and an ST-segment elevation occurs in VR as a 'mirror' image. (B) Schematic representation that explains how ST-segment depression is seen in all leads, except for VR and V1. The vector of circumferential subendocardial injury is directed from the subepicardium to the subendocardium and is seen as an ST depression in all the leads, except for VR and sometimes V1.

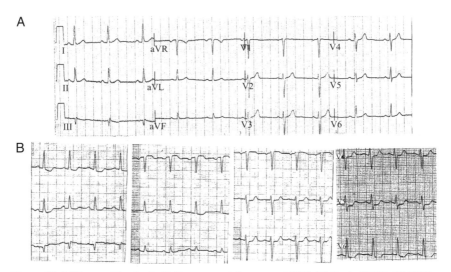

Figure 77 A 67-year-old patient with three-vessel disease and ACS. (A) Control ECG. (B) ECG during pain. See the ST depression in many leads with positive T wave in V4–V5, and slight ST elevation in VR and V1.

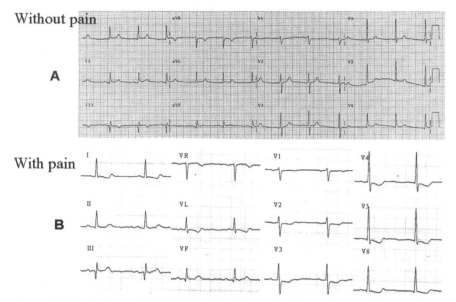

Figure 78 Patient with non-STE-ACS. The ECG without pain (A) is nearly normal. During pain, ST depression is left precordial leads and in some frontal leads with negative T waves in V4–V6. These cases correspond to non-STE-ACS with regional involvement of worst prognosis.

ACS with ST depression, even slight in less than 7 leads (**regional involvement**) with dominant R wave (Figures 78 and 79) or in leads with rS morphology (V1–V4), **present a worse prognosis than ACS with a new negative but usually not deep T wave** (Figure 80). One sub-study of GUSTO IIb trial [63] has demonstrated that cases of ST depression with **regional involvement** (less than 8 leads with ST depression) of worst prognosis correspond to cases with ST depression in V4–V6 and ST depression in I, VL or II, III, VF, especially if in V4–V6 there is negative T wave (two-to-three vessel disease) (Figure 78).

The group of NSTE-ACS that present flat/mild negative T wave (Figure 80) or even normal ECG, in the course of non STE-ACS usually has good prognosis. In case of doubt about the characteristics of pain it is compulsory to perform a very good differential diagnosis of precordial pain [57].

Other ST-segment deviations of ischaemic origin not due to a typical ACS

ST-segment elevation is usually found in coronary spasm (Prinzmetal angina) usually not related with ACS. The first ECG manifestation is often a peaked and tall T wave [45] (Figure 65). Occasionally an upward convex ST elevation, generally slight, may be persistent after the acute phase of a myocardial

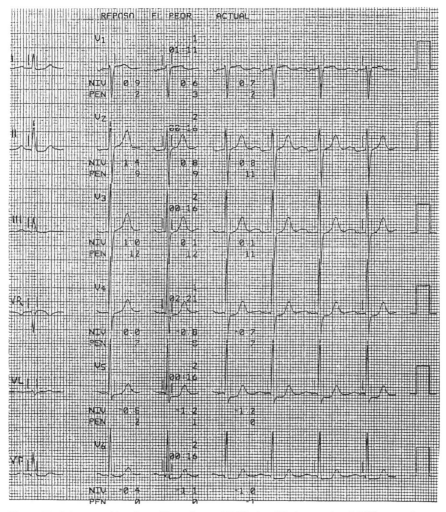

Figure 79 A 67-year-old patient with angina and ECG at rest that presents mild ST-segment depression. During exercise testing an increase of ST-segment depression ≥0.5 mm appeared with angina.

infarction. It is classically considered to be related to left ventricular aneurysm. The specificity of this sign is high, but its sensitivity is low. On the other hand, a slight ST-segment depression is frequently observed in coronary patients and is not necessarily related to the persistence of extensive ischaemia. If this is the case, it means that the ischaemia has a clear subendocardial predominance. If an exercise test may increase this pattern (≥1 mm) it usually represents true ischaemia (Figure 79).

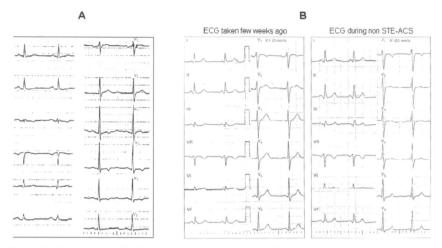

A

B

ECG taken few weeks ago

ECG during non STE-ACS

Figure 80 Two cases (A, B) of non-ST-segment elevation ACS with the negative T wave not present before the acute chest pain.

ST-segment deviations in conditions other than ischaemic heart disease

The most frequent causes of ST-segment elevation, apart from ischaemic heart disease, are displayed in Table 12. Figure 81 shows some of the most representative examples. With all these conditions, at the time of making the differential diagnosis, it is convenient to bear in mind in one's daily practice the pattern of the early phase of an acute pericarditis (Figures 82 and 83A), as it also occurs with chest pain that can confound the diagnosis, also with the pattern of vagal overdrive and early repolarisation.

Table 12 Most frequent causes of ST-segment elevation (apart from ischaemic heart disease).

1 **Normal variants.** Chest abnormalities, early repolarisation, vagal overdrive. In vagal overdrive, ST-segment elevation is mild, and generally accompanies the early repolarisation image. T wave is tall and asymmetric.

2 **Sportsmen.** Sometimes an ST-segment elevation exists that even mimics an acute infarction with or without negative T wave, at times prominent. No coronary involvement has been found, but this image has been observed in sportsmen who die suddenly; thus its presence implies the need to rule out hypertrophic cardiomyopathy.

3 **Acute pericarditis** in its early stage and myopericarditis.

4 **Pulmonary embolism.**

5 **Hyperkalaemia.** The presence of a tall peaked T wave is more evident than the accompanying ST-segment elevation, but sometimes it may be evident.

6 **Hypothermia.**

7 **Brugada's syndrome.**

8 **Arrhythmogenic right ventricular dysplasia.**

9 **Dissecting aortic aneurysm.**

10 **Left pneumothorax.**

11 **Toxicity secondary to cocaine abuse, drug abuse, etc.**

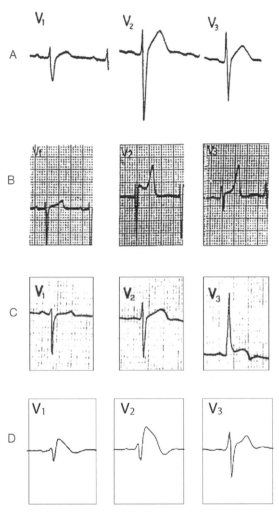

Figure 81 The most frequent cases of ST-segment elevation apart from ischaemic heart disease. (A) pericarditis; (B) hyperkaliemia; (C) athletes; (D) a typical Brugada pattern with coved ST-segment elevation. The saddle-type variant of Brugada syndrome has to be differentiated from normal variant (see Figures 22G and 105).

The most frequent causes of ST-segment depression in situations other that ischaemic heart disease are displayed in Table 13 and Figure 84.

Electrocardiographic pattern of necrosis

Electrocardiographic pattern of necrosis in the presence of normal cardiac activation

New concepts [46–60]

Classically, the electrocardiographic pattern of an established necrosis is associated with the presence of a **pathologic Q wave**, generally accompanied by a

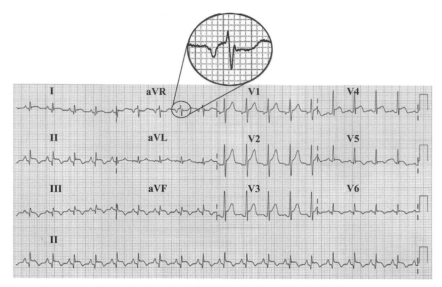

Figure 82 Patient with chest pain and small ST elevation in various leads. See the PR-segment elevation in VR that is in favour of atrial injury due to pericarditis.

negative T wave (necrosis Q wave) [46–48] (Table 14). This is the morphology seen both in the experimental animal model and also in clinical practice after total occlusion of a coronary artery with transmural involvement, after an initial phase of ST-segment elevation (Figure 85). Furthermore, until not so long ago it was thought that the cases of non-Q-wave infarction had a subendocardial

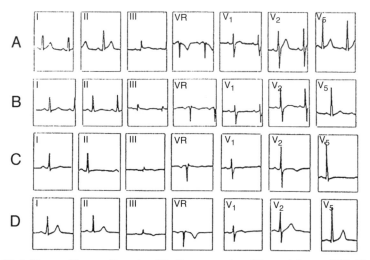

Figure 83 A 42-year-old man with pericarditis. Four examples of the evolutionary ECG. The A, B, C and D strips were recorded respectively on days 1, 8, 10 and 90 following onset of the event. (A) ST elevation is convex with respect to the isoelectrical line; (B) flattening of the T wave; (C) inversion of the T wave; and (D) normalisation.

Table 13 Most frequent causes of ST-segment depression (apart from ischaemic heart disease).

---

1 **Normal variants** (generally slight ST depression). Sympathetic overdrive. Neurocirculatory asthenia, hyperventilation, etc.
2 **Drugs** (diuretics, digitalis, etc.)
3 **Hypokalaemia**
4 **Mitral valve prolapse**
5 **Post-tachycardia**
6 **Secondary** to bundle branch block or ventricular hypertrophy. Mixed images are frequently generated.

---

location (electrically 'mute'). Thus, it was considered that Q-wave infarctions signified a transmural involvement, while the non-Q-wave infarctions implied a subendocardial compromise. However, we have to remember that there exist morphologies equivalent to a pathologic Q wave, such as the presence of a tall R wave in V1 (RS pattern). This pattern may be considered as equivalent of Q wave and may be observed in patients with evident, often transmural necrosis of the lateral wall (see Table 15). Significant advances have been made in recent years in understanding the ECG patterns of acute coronary syndromes and chronic infarctions [33–35,49,57]. The following are the most important:
• It is now well known that, from a clinical point of view, **isolated subendocardial infarctions usually do not exist**. Nevertheless, there are infarctions that compromise a great portion of the wall, but with subendocardial predominance, which may or may not develop a Q wave. Furthermore, there are completely transmural infarctions (such as the basal infarctions) that may not develop a Q wave and also the presence of second MI may cancel the presence of Q wave. This assumption has been recently confirmed by magnetic resonance studies. **Consequently, the distinction between transmural as equivalent to Q-wave infarctions and subendocardial equivalent to non-Q-wave infarctions can no longer be supported**.
• It is certain that **Q- and non-Q-wave infarctions** in the **subacute and chronic phases exist**, and we also have to remember that there exist some morphologies (see above) that are equivalent to Q wave as RS pattern in V1 as a mirror

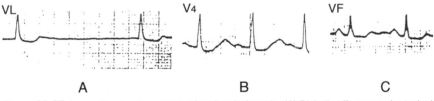

Figure 84 ST depression due to a cause other than ischaemia. (A) Digitalis effect: note the typical morphology with ST depression and short QT in a patient with slow atrial fibrillation; (B) hypokalemia in a patient with congestive heart failure taking high doses of furosemide; C) mitral valve prolapse.

Table 14 Characteristics of the 'necrosis Q wave' or its equivalent [1,21]*.

---

1 Duration: ≥30 ms in I, II, III[†], VL[‡] and VF, and in V3–V6. Frequently presents slurrings. The presence of a Q wave is normal in VR. In V1–V2, all Q waves are pathologic; Usually also in V3 except in the case of extreme levorotation (qRs in V3).
2 Q/R ratio: lead I and II > 25%, VL > 50%, V6 > 25% even in the presence of low R wave[†].
3 Depth: above the limit considered normal for each lead, i.e. generally 25% of the R wave (frequent exceptions, especially in VL, III and VF).
4 Presence of even a small Q wave in leads where it does not normally occur (for example, qrS in V1–V2).
5 Q wave with decreasing voltage from V3–V4 to V5–V6.
6 Equivalents of a Q wave in V1: R-wave duration ≥ 40 ms, and/or R-wave amplitude > 3 mm and/or R/S ratio > 0.5.

---

* The changes of mid-late part of QRS (low R wave and fractioned QRS) are not included in this list, which only mentions the changes of the first part of QRS (Q wave or equivalent).
[†] The presence of an isolated Q wave in lead III usually is non-pathologic. Check changes with inspiration. Usually in III and VF, QR ratios are not valuable when the voltage of R wave is low (< 5 mm).
[‡] QS morphology (⩒) may be seen in a normal heart in special circumstances (vertical heart).

image. Nevertheless, this simple distinction **does not permit differentiation between large and small infarctions although the presence of many Q waves means usually more extensive infarction than the existence of transmural involvement** [53]. Non-Q-wave infarctions, compared with Q-wave infarctions, show frequently more coronary arteries involved, a larger previous ischaemic area, more previous infarctions and a larger collateral circulation, but fewer total occlusions of the culprit coronary artery at the moment of the infarction.

• On the other hand, in patients with MI with or without Q waves, changes in the mid-late QRS morphology (rsr', slurrings) that correspond to the concept of **fractioned QRS** can be seen [54].

• However, in the acute phase the best classification of evolving infarction is ACS with ST elevation or without ST elevation because this implies specific management of the patient (fibrinolysis or early PCI, etc.).

• **In everyday practice** we still use the nomenclature of affected myocardial infarction zone according to the presence of Q waves in different leads as was proposed more than 50 years ago by Myers [57] on the basis of their classical pathological study. According to this classification, the presence of **Q wave in V1–V2 represents septal infarction, in V3–V4 anterior infarction, in V1–V4 anteroseptal infarction, in V5–V6 low lateral infarction, in V3–V6 anterolateral infarction, in V1–V6 anteroseptolateral infarction, in I and VL high lateral infarction, in II, III, VF inferior infarction, and the presence of RS in V1–V2 is explained by posterior infarction.** Nowadays, thanks to correlation with imaging techniques [51] including magnetic resonance [33–35,52] and with the knowledge of the electrophysiologic genesis of the first vector, we may affirm that the presence of Q wave in V1–V2 does not mean

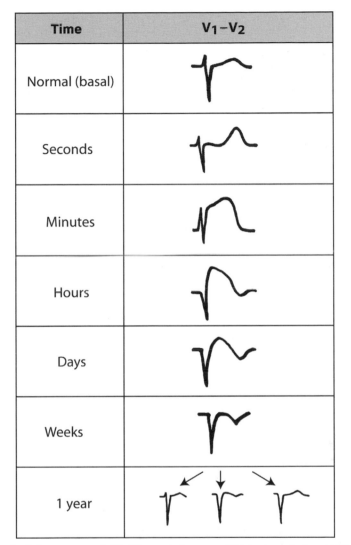

Time	V₁–V₂
Normal (basal)	
Seconds	
Minutes	
Hours	
Days	
Weeks	
1 year	

Figure 85 Evolutionary pattern in V1–V2 seen in the case of MI due to occlusion of LAD.

involvement of the entire septal wall, and that QS in V1–V4 does not mean that whole anteroseptal wall is involved [57]. As a matter of fact, the first vector of depolarisation is originated in the mid-low part of the anterior septum. Therefore, there is no need of involvement of the upper part of the septum for the appearance of Q wave in V1–V2. Obviously, if the LAD occlusion is very proximal (before S1 and D1) the high septum will be affected, but then Q waves in V5–V6, I and VL will be present due to occlusion proximal to the first diagonal (D1). Therefore, if Q wave is only present in precordials but not in

VL it is probable that the occlusion of the artery is in the mid-low part of LAD after first–second diagonal and also the first septal branches. This explains that myocardial infarctions with Q waves in precordials but not in I and VL are often not very extensive (apical MI) [51,52] and involve only the mid-low part of septum and anterior wall and usually also the apex because the LAD is long and wraps the apex (segment 17) [57].

• **The correlation between CMR and ECG patterns has allowed us to realize that there are seven ECG patterns that match very well with seven ECG areas of necrosis located in different areas of the left ventricle. This is the basis of our new classification of Q-wave MI that we will explain later on (Table 15)** [33–35].

• Finally, the **recent consensus** regarding the diagnosis of infarction **by the ESC/ACC** (European Society of Cardiology/American College of Cardiology) [49,50] accepts the diagnosis of infarction if troponin levels increase, accompanied by any of the other criteria listed in Table 15, not per se requiring the presence of electrocardiographic changes. Consequently, there are infarctions that involve less than the amount of necrotic tissue needed to modify the ECG [50]. This implies that many unstable anginas are turned into infarctions (microinfarctions or 'necrosettes'). Until this definition was accepted, it was uncommon to find a normal ECG in the acute stage of an infarction, and if it occurred it was due to small LCX or RCA artery occlusion.

Concept of Q-wave infarction

In Figure 85 we can observe the most frequent changes in the T wave, ST segment and QRS complex that appear in the evolutionary course of an acute coronary syndrome with ST-segment elevation evolving to a Q-wave myocardial infarction (Figure 85). Subendocardial ischaemia pattern—tall and peaked T wave (hyperacute phase)—followed by subepicardial injury pattern—ST elevation or equivalents—the Q wave of necrosis accompanied by the negative

---

Table 15 New criteria proposed for the diagnosis of infarction [49].

Either of the following two criteria is sufficient to establish the diagnosis of an evolving or recent acute infarction

1 Typical increase and gradual decrease in troponins levels* or other specific markers (CK-MB) of myocardial necrosis in the presence of at least one of the following:
   • Symptoms of ischaemia (angina or equivalent)
   • Development of pathologic Q waves in the ECG (Table 14)
   • Electrocardiographic changes indicative of ischaemia (ST-segment elevation or depression and or T wave inversion)
   • Interventional procedures in coronary arteries (e.g., PTCA)

2 Acute infarction anatomic-pathological changes

---

*It is convenient to remember the causes of a troponin increase in the absence of ischaemic heart disease, which include heart failure, renal failure, hypertensive crisis, etc.

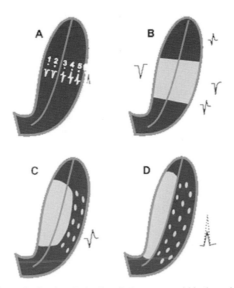

Figure 86 (A) Normal ventricular depolarisation; being very rapid in the subendocardium does not generate detectable potentials as this zone is very rich in Purkinje fibres (QS in 1 and 2). Starting from the border zone with subepicardium (3), morphologies with an increasing R wave (rS, RS, Rs) are registered (3 to 5) up to an exclusive R wave in epicardium (6). As a consequence, in the case of an experimental necrosis, the Q wave will be recorded only when it reaches subepicardium, as the vectors of necrosis will move away from the more necrotic area when this is more and more large. This originates qR morphology in 3, QR in 4 and 5, up to QS if the necrosis is transmural. (B) This explains how clinical transmural infarction originates QS morphology while (C) an infarction affecting subendocardium and a part of subepicardium may give rise to QR morphology without being necessarily transmural. Finally, (D) an infarction affecting subendocardium and a part of subepicardium, but in the form of patches, with necrosis-free zones, allows early formation of depolarisation vectors that will be recorded as R waves although of small voltage.

T wave of subepicardial ischemia appear in a sequential manner. Usually more than one of these patterns exist at the same time.

The STE-ACS usually evolves to a Q-wave MI that is often transmural (Figure 86B). However, a pathologic 'q' wave may be observed in non-transmural infarctions (Figure 86C) as well, and occasionally, a tall R wave instead of a pathologic 'Q' wave may be observed as it appears in V1–V2 leads as a mirror image, or a decrease of R wave voltage in V6 in the case of a transmural lateral or inferolateral infarction of basal areas or involving areas of subepicardium in form of patches (Figure 86D).

- Transmural infarction may be seen in patients with and without Q waves and the same may occur in cases of nontransmural infarction.
- The presence of Q wave is more a marker of extensive than transmural infarction.

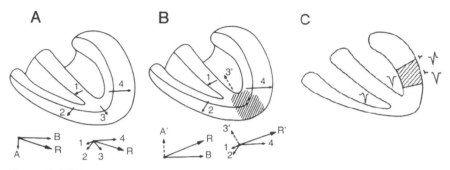

Figure 87 (A) Under normal conditions the global QRS vector (R) is formed by the sum of the different ventricular vectors (1+2+3+4). (B) When a necrotic zone exists, the corresponding vector (3 in the figure) has the same magnitude as before necrosis, but it is opposite in direction, determining modifications of the direction of the global vector (R′). (C) According to Wilson, the necrotic zone is an electric window that allows us to record the QS morphologies recorded in the left ventricular cavity.

Mechanisms of Q wave

The appearance of the Q wave of necrosis may be explained [1] by the **electrical window theory of Wilson** (Figure 87C) or by the formation of a **necrosis vector** with the corresponding loop (Figure 88A and B). The **vector of necrosis** is equal in magnitude, but opposite in direction, to the normal vector that would be generated in the same zone without necrosis. The onset of ventricular depolarisation changes when the necrotic area corresponds to a zone that

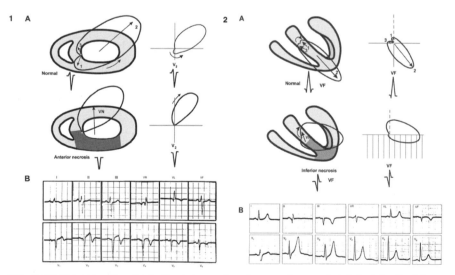

Figure 88 The necrosis vector is directed away from the necrotic zone. In inferior infarction it is directed upwards (1-A) and in the anterior infarction, backwards (2-A). See at the bottom (B) two examples of chronic myocardial infarction of anteroseptal and inferolateral zones.

is depolarised within the first 40 ms of ventricular activation, which occurs in a major part of the left ventricle except in the posterobasal parts.

Location and quantification of Q-wave myocardial infarction
Table 16 shows the correlation between leads with Q wave and area of myocardial necrosis detected by CMR and the most probable place of coronary occlusion responsible for MI [33–35]. However, in practice with new treatments of acute phase very often the coronariangiography performed in subacute or chronic phases usually shows a completely different coronary pattern because even in the case of established necrosis the coronary artery was lastly, at least partially, opened by treatment. We should bear in mind that the current treatment of acute coronary syndromes may lead to a reduction in infarct size (even 40–50%). Occasionally, an infarction may even be aborted and therefore usually there is a discrepancy between the presumed location of the occlusion and the final necrotic zone.

Figure 89 shows the old and new concepts of MI of the inferolateral zone, and Table 16 provides the new classification based on the concordance between Q-wave location in different leads and area involved detected by contrast-enhanced cardiovascular magnetic resonance (CE-CMR) correlations (global agreement 0.88%) [34,35]. Furthermore, the specificity of criteria of Q wave that we have used (see Table 14) is high and the sensitivity is also acceptable, although it is lower especially in the case of mid-anterior and lateral MI (Table 16).

A quantitative QRS score system was developed by Selvester [55] to estimate extension of myocardial necrosis especially in the case of myocardial infarction of the anterior zone. The most significant number of mistakes was due to the fact that the score system considered that Q wave in V1–V2 implies septal involvement including the basal area. As we have already stated, this is not true because the first vector (r in V1–V2) is generated in the mid-low anterior part of the septum, but not in the basal part. **In spite of the global value of this score to estimate the involved mass, currently the CE-CMR gives us a much more exact measurement of chronic infarcted area in a particular case** [53,56,57].

Examples of seven ECG patterns in the case of myocardial infarction of inferolateral and anteroseptal zones and its location detected by CE-CMR are shown in Figures 90–96. The infarcted areas are in white, due to the retention of gadolinium in these areas (see Table 16). The planes of the heart in the CMR images are explained in the figure legends, according to Figure 55 (see also Table 16).

Differential diagnosis of pathologic Q wave
The specificity of the pathologic Q wave for diagnosing a myocardial infarction is high, especially in adults older than 40 years. Nevertheless, we should bear in mind that similar or the same Q waves can be seen in other conditions. We should remember that the diagnosis of myocardial infarction is based not only

Table 16 Location of Q wave.

	Name	Type	ECG pattern	Infarction area (CE-CMR)	Most probable place of occlusion
Anteroseptal, zone	Septal	A1	Q in V1–V2 SE: 100% SP: 97%		LAD
	Apical–anterior	A2	Q in V1–V2 to V3–V6 SE: 85% SP: 98%		LAD
	Extensive anterior	A3	Q in V1–V2 to V4–V6, I and aVL SE: 83% SP: 100%		LAD
	Mid-anterior	A4	Q (qs or qr) in aVL (I) and sometimes in V2–V3 SE: 67% SP: 100%		LAD
Inferolateral, zone	Lateral	B1	RS in V1–V2 and/or Q wave in leads I, aVL, V6 and/or diminished R wave in V6 SE: 67% SP: 99%		LCX
	Inferior	B2	Q in II, III, aVF SE: 88% SP: 97%		RCA LCX
	Inferolateral	B3	Q in II, III, Vf (B2) and Q in I, VL, V5–V6 and/or RS in V1 (B1) SE: 73% SP: 98%		RCA LCX

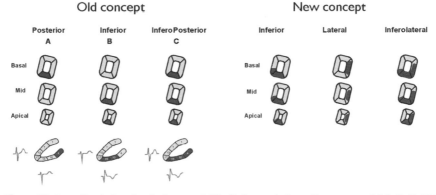

Figure 89 According to the classical concept, MI of inferoposterior wall may present Q in II, III, VF (inferior MI), or RS in V1–V2 (posterior MI). The presence of both criteria is seen in the case of inferoposterior MI. If the MI also encompasses the lateral wall the only ECG new criterion may be the presence of abnormal Q wave in lateral leads or very low R in V6. Currently, the MI of interolateral zone may be clustered in three groups: Q in II, III, VF (inferior MI with or without the involvement of the inferobasal segment – old posterior wall); RS in V1 and/or abnormal 'q' in lateral leads (lateral MI). Inferolateral MI encompasses both criteria (see Figure 59).

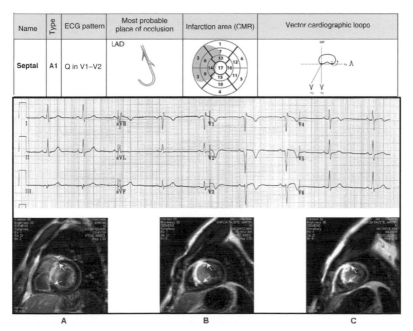

Figure 90 Example of large septal MI (type A-1) ECG criteria (Q in V1–V2 with rS in V3), most probable site of occlusion, CE-CMR images and VCG loops. The septal infraction is very extensive encompassing the greatest part of the septal wall less the most interior, at all levels—basal (A), mid (B) and apical (C) on transverse plane. There is small extension towards the anterior wall at mid and apical levels (arrows).

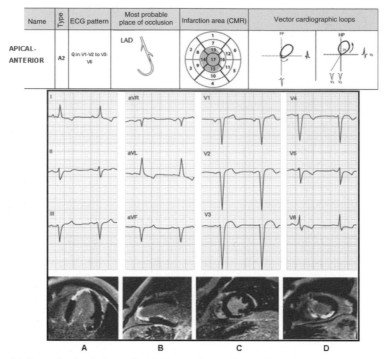

Name	Type	ECG pattern	Most probable place of occlusion	Infarction area (CMR)	Vector cardiographic loops
APICAL-ANTERIOR	A2	Q in V1-V2 to V3-V6	LAD		

Figure 91 Example of apical-anterior MI (Q wave beyond V_2). In the horizontal plane (A) the septal and apical involvement is seen. The sagital plane (B) shows that the inferior involvement is even larger than the anterior involvement, and in the mid and low transverse transections, especially in D, the septal and inferior involvement is seen.

on electrocardiographic alterations but also on clinical evaluation and enzymatic changes. The pattern of ischaemia or injury accompanying a pathologic Q wave supports the idea that the Q wave is secondary to ischaemic heart disease. However, in 5–25% of Q-wave infarctions (with the highest incidence in inferior infarction) the Q wave disappears with time, therefore its sensitivity for detecting old myocardial infarction is not high. The main causes of pathological Q wave due to causes other than myocardial necrosis are listed in Table 17.

Myocardial infarction without Q wave

Table 18 shows different types of myocardial infarctions without Q wave. The most typical is the **non-Q-wave infarction**. In this case, diagnosis should be based on the presence of typical clinical symptoms of acute ischaemia accompanied by enzymatic changes and repolarisation alterations (ST and/or negative T wave) and sometimes the presence of **fractioned QRS** (notches and slurring in mid–late QRS complex) but without necrotic Q wave appearance. Figure 70 shows the evolutive changes that frequently appear in the case of

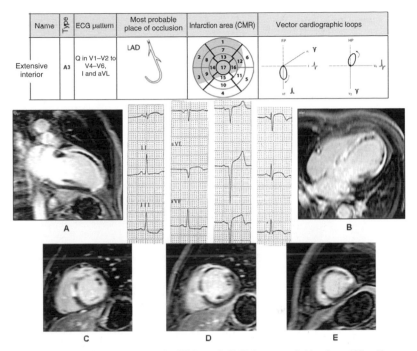

Figure 92 Example of extensive anterior MI (type A-3) (Q in precordial leads and VL with qrs in L). Most probable place of occlusion, CE-CMR image and the VCG loops of this case. CE-CMR images show the extensive involvement of septal, anterior and lateral walls, less the highest part of the lateral wall (see B and C). The involvement of segments 7 and 12 explain that in this MI there is a Q in VL that is not present in MI of apical–anterior-type (A). Oblique sagittal view (B). Longitudinal horizontal plane view and C to E. Transverse view. The inferior wall is the only spared. The LAD is not very large and therefore the inferior involvement is not extensive (see A). Due to that there is QS in aVL and R in II, III and aVF together with Q in VI to V5.

non-Q-wave MI. The incidence of myocardial infarctions without Q wave increases as some ACS with ST elevation do not develop Q wave due to thrombolytic treatment. The prognosis is worse when signs of residual ischaemia exist.

Diagnosis of necrosis in the presence of ventricular blocks, pre-excitation or pacemaker

Complete right bundle branch block (Figure 97)

In the **chronic phase**, since cardiac activation begins normally the presence of an infarction causes an alteration in the first part of the QRS complex that can generate a necrosis Q wave, just as in the cases with normal ventricular conduction. Furthermore, in the **acute phase** the ST–T changes can be seen as in the cases with normal activation. Patients with an acute coronary syndrome

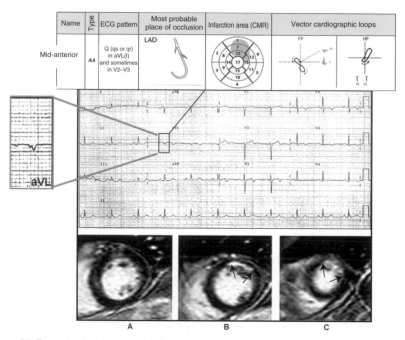

Figure 93 Example of mid-anterior MI (type A-4) (QS in VL without Q in V5–6), most probable place of occlusion, CE-CMR image and the VCG loop in this case. CE-CMR images shows in transverse plane mid-low-anterior and lateral wall involvement (B,C).

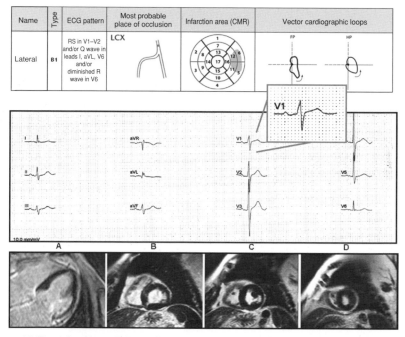

Figure 94 Example of lateral MI with RS in V1 (type B-1). See the most probable place of occlusion, the CE-CMR image and the VCG loops. The CE-CMR images show that in this case the MI involves especially the basal and mid part of the lateral wall (A–C) (longitudinal horizontal and transverse planes) but not the apical part (D).

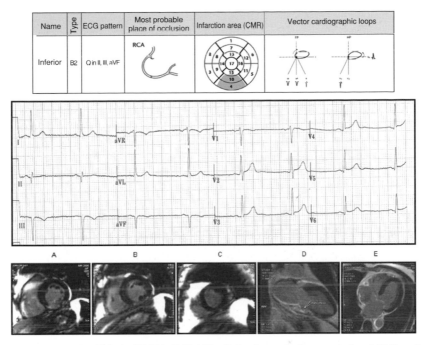

Figure 95 Example of inferior MI (Q in II, III, VF) with involvement of segments 4 and 10 (A and D), and rS morphology in V1. There is no lateral and septal involvement (E).

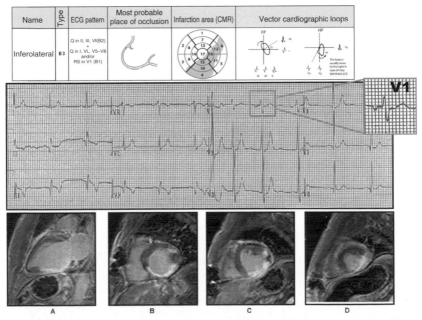

Figure 96 Example of inferolateral MI (Q in II, III, VF and RS in V1). The most probable place of occlusion (RCA), the CE-CMR image and the corresponding VCG loops. The CMR images show the involvement of inferior wall and also part of lateral wall. (A) Saggital-like transection showing the involvement of inferior wall. (B–D) Transverse transections at basal, mid and apical level showing also the lateral involvement especially seen on mid and apical level.

Table 17 Pathologic Q wave not secondary to myocardial infarction.

1. During the evolution of an acute disease involving the heart
    1.1. Acute coronary syndrome with an aborted infarction
    1.2. Coronary spasm (Prinzmetal angina type)
    1.3. Acute myocarditis
    1.4. Presence of transient apical dyskinesia that also shows ST-segment elevation and a transient pathologic 'q' wave. Probably corresponds to an aborted infraction: Tako–tsubo syndrome.
    1.5. Pulmonary embolism
    1.6. Miscellaneous: toxic agents, etc.
2. Chronic pattern
    2.1. Recording artefacts
    2.2. Normal variants: VL in the vertical heart and III in the dextrorotated and horizontalised heart
    2.3. QS in V1 (hardly ever in V2) in septal fibrosis, emphysema, the elderly, chest abnormalities, etc.
    2.4. Some types of right ventricular hypertrophy (chronic cor pulmonale) or left ventricular hypertrophy (QS in V1–V2), or slow increase in R wave in precordial leads, or abnormal 'q' wave in hypertrophic cardiomyopathy, sometimes deep but narrow and usually with normal repolarisation
    2.5. Left bundle branch conduction abnormalities
    2.6. Infiltrative processes (amyloidosis, sarcoidosis, tumours, chronic myocarditis, dilated cardiomyopathy, etc.)
    2.7. Wolff–Parkinson–White syndrome
    2.8. Congenital heart diseases (coronary artery abnormalities, dextrocardia)
    2.9. Pheochromocytoma

Table 18 Myocardial infarction without Q wave or equivalents.

1 **Non-Q wave infarction**
   • ST-segment depression and/or negative T wave: new ST ≥ 0.5 mm or new flat or negative T wave.
   • Sometimes with the presence of changes in mid-late QRS (fractioned QRS).
2 **Infarctions located in areas that do not originate Q wave of necrosis**
   a Atria (an isolated location never exists): infarction is usually present in an extensive area.
   b Basal segments: often secondary to the occlusion of a non-proximal LCX or RCA (sometimes with fractioned QRS).
   c Right ventricle (usually does not present isolated): it is accompanied by an inferior infarction. It is secondary to occlusion of a proximal RCA before the take-off of the right ventricle marginal branches.
   d Microinfarction (enzymatic).
5 **Aborted Q wave**
   • Acute coronary syndrome with ST-segment elevation (evolving infarction) but with quite early and efficient reperfusion. troponins levels will tell us whether it is an unstable angina or a non-Q-wave infarction.
6 **Q of infarctions that disappear during the follow-up**
7 **Masked Q wave**
   • Ventricular block;
   • Wolff—Parkinson—White;   } May sometimes show a pathologic Q wave.
   • Pacemakers.

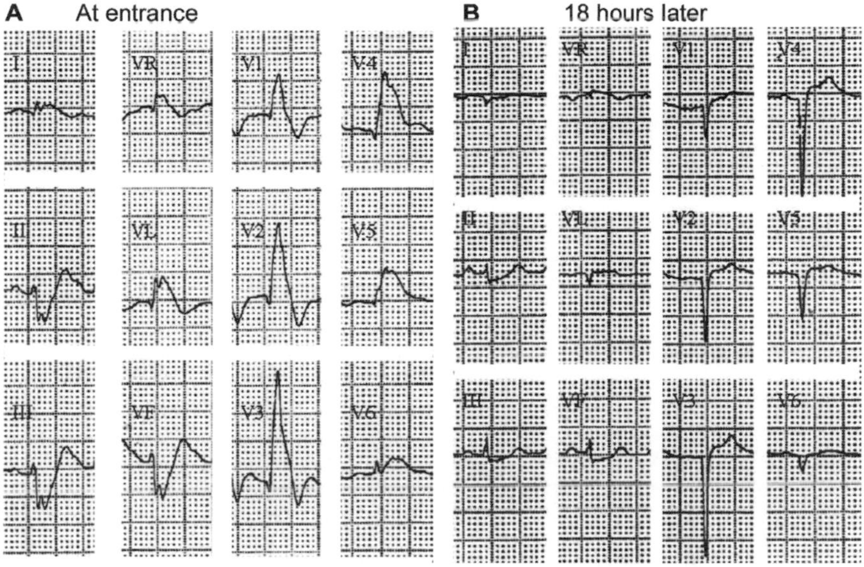

A   At entrance

B   18 hours later

Figure 97 A typical example of RBBB plus acute MI of anteroseptal zone.

with ST elevation, which in its course shows a complete new-onset right bundle branch block, usually have the LAD occluded before the first septal and first diagonal. This is explained by the fact that the right bundle branch receives perfusion from S1.

Complete left bundle branch block (Figure 98)

In the acute phase, the diagnosis of myocardial infarction in the presence of a complete left bundle branch block may be suggested by specific ST-segment deviations (any ST elevation or huge ST depression in case of R morphology, and any ST depression or huge ST elevation in case of rS morphology [58]).

In the chronic phase, ventricular depolarisation starts in the part proximal to the base of the anterior papillary muscle of the right ventricle. This generates a depolarisation vector (vector 1) directed forwards, downwards and to the left. Subsequently, transseptal depolarisation of the left ventricle generates vectors 2, 3 and 4. As a result, even if important zones of the left ventricle are necrotic the overall direction of the depolarisation vector does not change, and these vectors continue to point from right to left, impeding inscription of a Q necrosis wave. Nevertheless, evident 'q' waves in I, V6 or tall R waves in V1 may be occasionally observed (Figure 98). The correlation of clinical and ECG changes with enzymatic changes and changes in radionuclide studies [59] confirmed that the presence of Q waves in I, VL, V5, V6 and R in V1–V2 leads is the most specific criterion for diagnosing myocardial infarction in the presence of a left bundle branch block in the chronic phase.

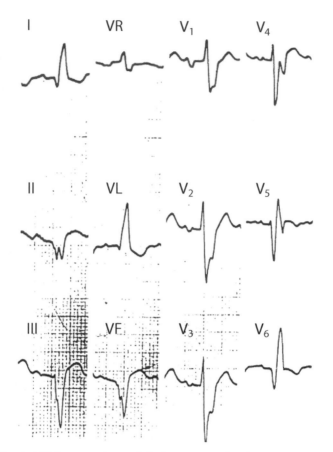

Figure 98 A typical ECG pattern of necrosis in the presence of a left bundle branch block. Observe the pathologic 'Q' wave in I, VL and V6, 'r' wave in V1 and polyphasic morphology in V4–V5.

Hemiblocks

In general, necrosis associated with the **superoanterior hemiblock** may be diagnosed without problems. Usually, we may assess in the case of ECG with left AQRS deviation and Q wave in II, III, VF whether the myocardial infarction is isolated or associated with the **superoanterior hemiblock** (SAH). The loop–hemifield correlations explain that in the absence of SAH in lead II there is Qr morphology and in its presence the morphology is an isolated QS pattern especially of W type (Figures 99 A and B). In some cases, mainly in small inferior infarctions, the superoanterior hemiblock may mask myocardial necrosis. The initial vector (vector 1) is directed more downwards than normal as a result of SAH and masks a necrosis vector of small inferior infarction (Figure 99C). The **inferoposterior hemiblock (IPH)** may mask or decrease the inferior necrosis pattern by converting QS or Qr morphology in II, III and VF into QR or qR (Figure 100). It may also originate a small positivity in I and VL in the case

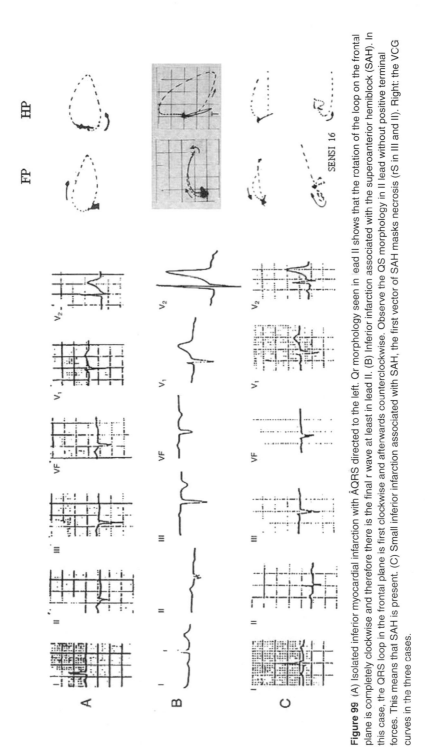

FP   HP

SENSI 16

Figure 99 (A) Isolated inferior myocardial infarction with ÂQRS directed to the left. Qr morphology seen in ead II shows that the rotation of the loop on the frontal plane is completely clockwise and therefore there is the final r wave at least in lead II. (B) Inferior infarction associated with the superoanterior hemiblock (SAH). In this case, the QRS loop in the frontal plane is first clockwise and afterwards counterclockwise. Observe the QS morphology in II lead without positive terminal forces. This means that SAH is present. (C) Small inferior infarction associated with SAH, the first vector of SAH masks necrosis (rS in III and II). Right: the VCG curves in the three cases.

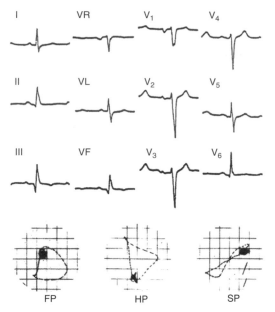

Figure 100 The ECG and VCG curves in a patient with inferior myocardial infarction associated with the inferoposterior hemiblock (IPH). See Rs in I and qR in II, III, and AVF, with a very open loop suggestive of the associated IPH.

of lateral infarction because the initial vector (vector 1 in the case of IPH) is directed more upwards than usual as a result of IPH and mask the necrosis vector of small lateral infarction.

Pre-excitation and pacemakers

It is difficult to diagnose the association of myocardial infarction in the presence of **pre-excitation**. Sometimes it may be suggested by evident changes of repolarisation especially in the acute phase of ACS.

Also in patients with pacemakers the changes in repolarisation, especially ST elevation, may suggest ACS [60]. In the chronic phase the presence of a spike-qR pattern, especially in V5–V6, is highly specific but little sensitive sign of necrosis.

CHAPTER 12

Miscellaneous

Value of ECG in special conditions [1,5,21]

The most characteristic ECG patterns of different special clinical conditions as ionic imbalance (A), hypothermia (B) and athletics (C) are shown in Figures 101–103 (see legends). Athletes may present first and even second degree AV block of vagal origin and also rSr' in V1 due to delay of activation of right ventricular and sometimes some degree of right ventricular enlargement (see Case 22).

ECG pattern of poor prognosis

Figures 104–106 show the most characteristic ECG patterns of genetically induced conditions such as long QT syndrome (Figure 104), Brugada's syndrome (Figure 105) and arrhythmogenic right ventricular dysplasia (Figure 106). The most characteristic features of ECG in hypertrophic cardiomyopathy are striking signs of LV enlargement and the presence of abnormal 'q' wave (see section 'Left ventricular enlargement' in Chapter 8 and Table 17).

ECG of electrical alternans [1] (Figure 107, Table 19)

Alternans of ECG morphologies signifies the repetitive and alternans change in the morphology of the QRS complex, ST segment or, rarely, P wave. The presence of certain changes in QRS morphology during sinus rhythm may occasionally be observed in precordial leads, particularly in very thin persons during respiration. **True alternans of QRS complexes (change in morphology without change of width) in patients with sinus rhythm is suggestive of cardiac tamponade** (Figure 107A). Alternans of QRS morphology may also be observed during **supraventricular arrhythmias, especially in patients with WPW.** Nevertheless, **true alternans** of QRS complexes can be confounded with QRS changes appearing in the form of bigeminy such as alternans bundle branch block, alternans WPW and ventricular bigeminy with very late ventricular ectopic beats (in the PR). In these situations, two clearly distinct QRS-T morphologies exist with different QRS width and sometimes with changes in the PR interval.

Alternans of ST–T may be observed in the **hyperacute phase of severe myocardial ischaemia** (Figure 107B), in the **congenital long QT syndrome** and in significant **electrolytic imbalance** (Figure 107C).

Recently, **T-wave alternans detected by microvoltage techniques has been found to be a marker of poor prognosis in post-MI patients and patients with other heart diseases.**

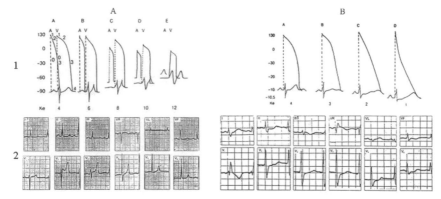

Figure 101 (1A) ECG alterations observed in successive stages of hyperkalemia. The atrial and ventricular action potential has been superimposed. With the increase of Ke, the level of DTP, height of Phase 0, and its rate of rise (the points of the dotted line are closer together) are all decreased. The surface ECG shows that the QRS duration is increased and the P wave disappears (adapted from [64]). (2A) A 20-year-old male with chronic renal failure who had periodic hemodialysis during the 2 years prior to the recording. There is severe hypertension (210/130 mmHg) and an elevated potassium level (6.4 mEq/L). Note the tall and peaked T wave and elevation of the ST segment in V2 and V3. In leads I, II, and III, QT is relatively long at the expense of the ST segment due to associated hypocalcemia. (1B) ECG alterations observed in successive stages of hypokalemia. The ventricular action potential has been superimposed. On the left is the DTP value, and below, the Ke level. Note how the action potential duration progressively increases at the expense of a decrease in the velocity of phase 2. The ECG shows a progressively bigger U wave and lesser T wave, together with an evident descent of the ST segment (adapted from [64]). (2B) A 45-year-old patient with advanced mitro-aortic valve disease who was treated with excessive doses of digitalis and diuretics. The Ke value is 2.3 mEq/L. An ECG alteration representing phase C (above) is clearly seen, particularly in V2–V4.

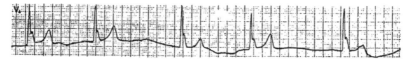

Figure 102 The ECG in the case of hypothermia. See the Osborne wave at the end of QRS, the presence of bradycardia and the oscillatory QRS baseline.

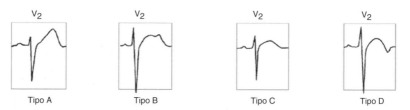

Figure 103 The four most evident repolarisation abnormalities found in athletes without evidence of heart disease. However, it is necessary to take a thorough history and often an echocardiogram and an effort test to rule out any heart diseases (hypertonic cardiomiopathy, coronary heart disease, etc.).

Figure 104 The typical ECG patterns in the case of long QT syndrome related to genetic alterations in chromosomes 3, 7 and 11.

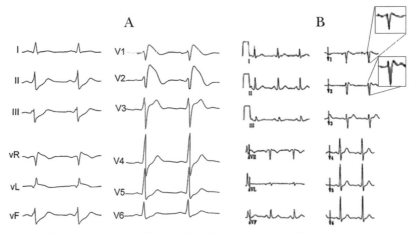

Figure 105 The Brugada pattern. On the left (A) is the typical one with the typical coved ST-segment elevation and on the right (B) the more difficult to recognise with r′ and saddle pattern elevation of ST. In the atypical Brugada pattern usually the r′ is wider than in the case of pectus excavatus (see Figure 22G) or athletes [61].

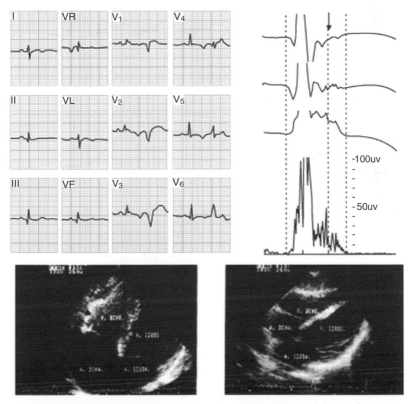

Figure 106 Arrhythmogenic right ventricular dysplasia (ARVD). Note the image of atypical right bundle branch block, negative T wave in the V1–V4 leads, and premature ventricular complexes of the right ventricle with left bundle branch block morphology. QRS duration is much longer in V1–V2 than in V6. On the right very positive late potentials are seen in the signal averaging ECG. Below: a typical echocardiographic image of right ventricle dyskinesia (see the arrow) in a patient with ARVD.

Table 19 Most frequent causes of QRS-T alternans.

QRS complex alternans
Rarely in relation with respiration especially in mid-precordial leads
Cardiac tamponade
Supraventricular arrhythmias in WPW syndrome

ST–T alternans
Hyperacute phase of severe myocardial ischaemia
Congenital long QT syndrome
Electrolytic imbalance

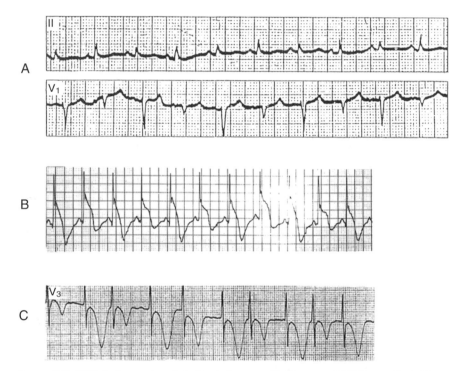

Figure 107 (A) Typical examples of electrical alternans. (A) Alternans of QRS in a patient with pericardial tamponade. (B) ST–QT alternans in Prinzmetal angina. (C) Repolarisation alternans in important electrolyte imbalance.

Self-assessment

To confirm whether you have understood the book and to check your ECG interpretative skills, we will proceed by conducting a multiple-choice test. In this test, you will be asked to give a correct answer based on presented ECG recordings. The examples of ECG tracings are based on the contents displayed in the book.

The correct answers as well as comments and explanations will be given.

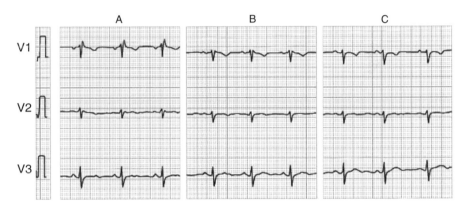

Case 1

A young, asthenic man with no apparent heart disease. The figure shows an ECG tracing in V1, V2 and V3 leads located in the second (A), third (B) and fourth (C) intercostal space. What is the correct diagnosis?

A Atrial septal defect
B Partial right bundle branch block
C Brugada's syndrome
D False image of right bundle branch block

Answer to Case 1

Comment. (A) Normal ECG recording, except V1, where final R wave is quite prominent and final r in V2 and RS morphology in V3 are present. Due to this morphology in V1 it is necessary to rule out RBBB. The evidence that the P wave in V1 is completely negative made us think that V1 lead is placed higher (second right intercostal space) and is recording the tail of the P vector (negative P) and the head of the third vector of ventricular depolarisation (terminal R). The lower location of the lead (B) decreased this image and it totally disappeared (positive P wave and rS in V1) when the lead was located correctly in fourth right intercostal space (C). We can conclude that in this case a false pattern of RBBB is present due to incorrect position of V1–V2 leads. The correct answer is D. Occasionally, the Brugada syndrome can present similar morphologies to 'A' and also the morphology may change depending on the lead position; but in the Brugada pattern the r′ in V1 is wider and ST-segment elevation in V1–V2 is present (see Table 4).

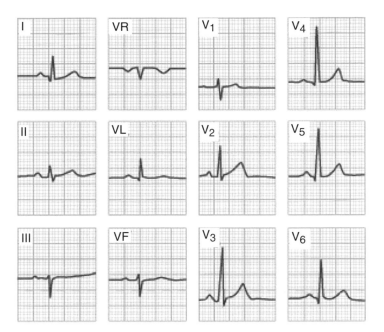

Case 2

A 27-year-old man with no apparent heart disease. What is the correct diagnosis?

A Acute pericarditis

B Early repolarisation in a subject with a horizontal heart with levorotation

C Acute phase of a myocardial infarction

D Dextrorotated heart

Answer to Case 2

Comment. There is important levorotation (Rs in V2) with mild ST-segment elevation starting from the J point, visible in V2–V4. This pattern corresponds to the so-called early repolarisation pattern. In the frontal plane with horizontal heart we can see qR in VL and rS in VF with ÂQRS approximately −15° and in the horizontal plane levorotation is present (Rs in V2 and qR in V4). The exercise test normalises the ST-segment elevation in the early repolarisation pattern as it happened in this case, but not in acute pericarditis or the acute phase of MI. Thus, the correct answer is B (see Figures 22D and 25-2a).

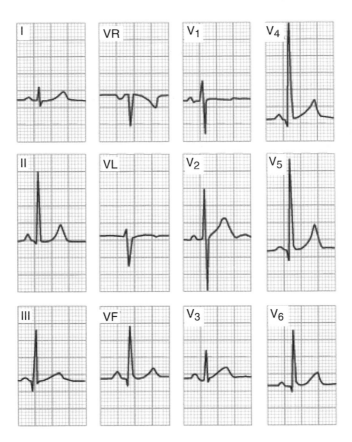

Case 3

An 18-year-old lean man, asymptomatic, with no heart disease. What is the correct diagnosis?

A Left ventricular enlargement

B Normal ECG variant; vertical heart with apparent levorotation

C Normal ECG variant; horizontal heart

D Normal ECG; heart with no rotation

Answer to Case 3

Comment. Vertical heart but without dextrorotation (there is no S in V5–V6). On the contrary, it seems that there is levorotation, as large R (Rs) in V2–V3 is seen. This can be explained knowing that in lean individuals with a long and narrow thorax, the heart is located more in the centre of the thorax and V3 already faces the left ventricle. ST-segment elevation in V2–V3 from the early repolarisation type (asymmetric T wave) is seen. The high voltage of the R wave in V4 is striking (>30 mm). This value is higher than the accepted as normal for adults, but can be observed in teenagers without heart disease and with normal echocardiogram, as it is in this case. Thus, the correct answer is B (see Figures 22D and 25.1A).

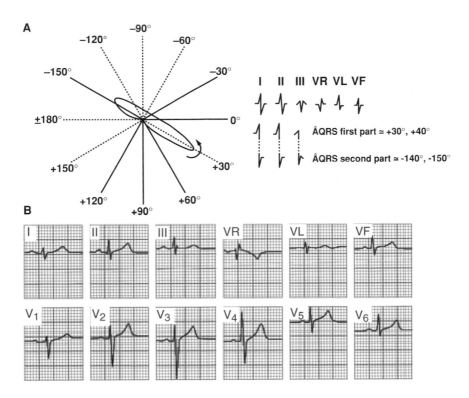

Case 4

A 28-year-old very lean man, with slight *pectus excavatum*, but with no apparent heart disease. What is the correct diagnosis?

A Right ventricular enlargement
B Normal heart with rotation on transversal axis (S_I, S_{II}, S_{III})
C Superoanterior hemiblock
D Vertical heart

Answer to Case 4

Comment. ECG recording with S_I S_{II} S_{III} morphologies in the frontal plane. Similar morphologies can be seen in right ventricular enlargement and, probably, in the right superoanterior zonal block (see Table 6). The absolutely normal appearance of the P and T waves supports a normal heart with rotation type S_I, S_{II}, S_{III} (transversal axis) (p. 26). The presence of RS in V5–V6 is due to additional dextrorotation. The extreme left deviation of ÂQRS, in the case of superoanterior hemiblock, generates morphologies with S_{II} and S_{III} but with $S_{III} > S_{II}$, on the contrary, that in this case (see Figure 43B). The normal clinical observation of the patient, including the echocardiography and the absence of pulmonary involvement, also the age and the presence of pectus excavatum, together with the normal P and T waves, supports the diagnosis of the normal heart with rotation on the transversal axis. The vertical heart presents RS in I and qR in II and III. Above: the QRS loop in such cases and the method of ÂQRS calculation from the first and the second part of QRS. Thus, the correct answer is B (see p. 26 and Figure 43B).

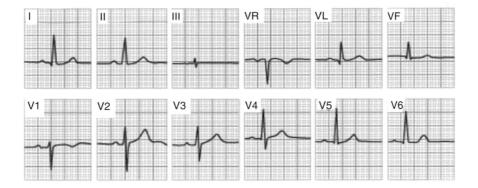

Case 5

A 35-year-old man with no apparent heart disease. What is the correct diagnosis?

A Heart with no apparent rotation
B Vertical heart
C Horizontal heart
D Indeterminate electrical axis

Answer to Case 5

Comment. ECG of a heart without apparent rotations. ÂQRS at +30° (rs in III and qR in VL and VF). The rest of the recording is in the normal range. ÂP = 0°, ÂT = + 30°. Thus, the correct answer is A (see p. 26 and Figure 24A).

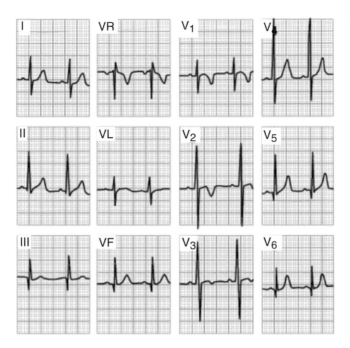

Case 6

A 6-year-old child with no apparent heart disease. What is the correct diagnosis?

A Normal ECG
B Right ventricular overload
C Left ventricular enlargement
D Pericarditis

Answer to Case 6

Comment. Normal ECG for the age of the patient. Observe the right ÂQRS, the relatively tall R wave in V1 greater than 'q' in V6, the R wave of large voltage in V4–V5, the deep 'q' wave in III, the infantile repolarisation, etc. The ECG is normal. Thus, the correct answer is A (see p. 30 and Figure 27A).

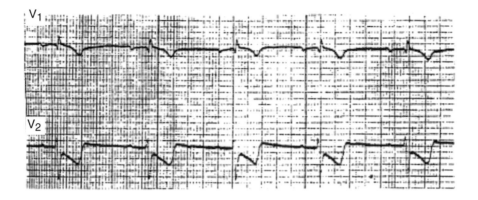

Case 7

These are leads V1 and V2 of a 60-year-old woman with a heart disease. Which is the correct diagnosis?

A Lateral myocardial infarction
B Significant enlargement of right cavities
C Complete right bundle branch block
D Type-II Wolff–Parkinson–White syndrome

Answer to Case 7

Comment. This ECG belongs to a 60-year-old patient with a long-standing mitral and tricuspid valve disease, with a significant right ventricle and atrial enlargement (see the low-voltage qR pattern in V1 and the rS pattern in V2 with a much higher voltage). The patient was in atrial fibrillation, with not visible 'f' waves. Spontaneously, she converted to normal sinus rhythm with a P wave that was only visible, but quite small, in V1–V2. Most probably, the presence of a significant atrial fibrosis could explain that large atria, as demonstrated in the echocardiographic study, generate a barely visible voltage in the surface ECG. Occasionally, even normal sinus rhythm can be completely concealed. The ECG does not show the presence of a complete right bundle branch block, as the QRS complex is narrow, nor does it show the presence of a Wolff–Parkinson–White syndrome, as the PR segment is not short, nor does it suggest the presence of a lateral infarction, as the morphology is not that of an R or Rs complex with a positive T wave, but of a qR complex with a negative T wave. Therefore, the correct answer is B (see p. 35 and p. 40).

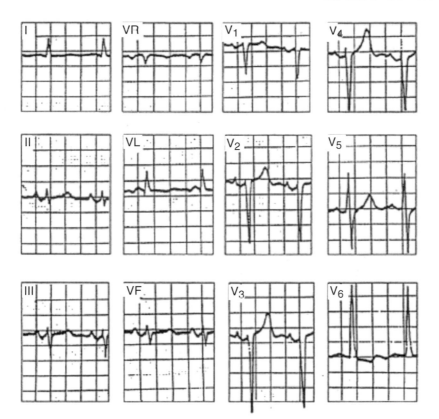

Case 8

This is a 45-year-old patient suffering from a heart disease, with the diagnosis having been made 30 years ago. Which is the correct diagnosis?

A Significant left ventricular and atrial enlargement
B Complete left bundle branch block
C Superoanterior hemiblock
D Acute septal infarction

Answer to Case 8

Comment. This is a patient with a valvular heart disease presenting a significant left ventricular enlargement (LVE), with a pure R wave in lead V6 with a systolic overload pattern and an S wave in V2 + an R wave in V6 = 45 mm. The P wave is wide and ± in leads II, III and VF, and from V1 to V4. It corresponds to a typical complete interatrial block with left atrium retrograde conduction that is always associated with left atrial enlargement. Therefore, the correct answer is A. The other diagnoses can be ruled out. (1) Complete left bundle branch block: the QRS complex is not equal to or longer than 0.12 seconds. (2) Superoanterior hemiblock: ÂQRS is not beyond −45°. (3) Acute septal infarction: there is no QS complex in V1–V2, and the ST-segment elevation, which is convex with respect to the isoelectric baseline, may be explained as a mirror image of the LVE morphology that is seen in V6 (see p. 37 and p. 44).

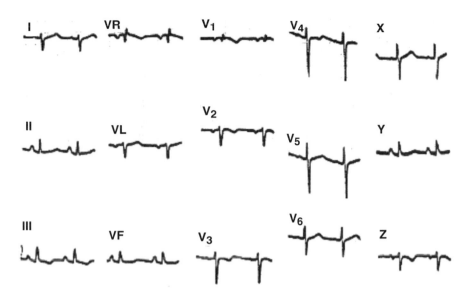

Case 9

This is a 65-year-old patient. The history taking is normal, with antecedents of chronic obstructive pulmonary disease dating back more than 20 years (recently with an acute crisis). Which is the correct diagnosis?

A Right ventricular and atrial enlargement

B Complete right bundle branch block

C Acute coronary syndrome with a negative T wave from V1 to V3

D Normal variant (vertically orientated heart) with no associated disease

Answer to Case 9

Comment. The 12-lead ECG and the orthogonal ECG (X, Y, Z, similar to I, VF and V2) of a 65-year-old patient with a chronic obstructive pulmonary disease (COPD). Note the presence of a rightward ÂQRS (> +90°), a qr pattern in V1 with an rS pattern in V6 as signs of right ventricular enlargement (RVE). The rightward ÂP with peaked P waves in leads II, III and VF, with relatively high voltage if it is to be compared with the QRS complex, is a sign suggestive of a right atrial enlargement (RAE). The P wave is negative in V1 as is frequently the case in COPD as, given that the ÂP is in quite a vertical position, its projection on the horizontal plane (HP) is minimal and, additionally, it can fall into the negative hemifield of lead V1. Note the similarity between orthogonal leads X, Y, Z with leads I, VF and V2 in the surface ECG. These signs are not compatible with a normal variant. On the other hand, T-wave morphology from V1 to V4 can be explained by the right chamber overload produced by the COPD and not by anteroseptal ischaemia due to an acute coronary syndrome. Nor are complete right bundle branch block electrocardiographic signs found: a QRS of less than 0.12 seconds and the V1 morphology with an r′ wave in V1 that could be explained by the RVE, even when its origin is partly due to a delay in the stimulus conduction within the right ventricle (RV). Therefore, the correct answer is A (see p. 35 and p. 41).

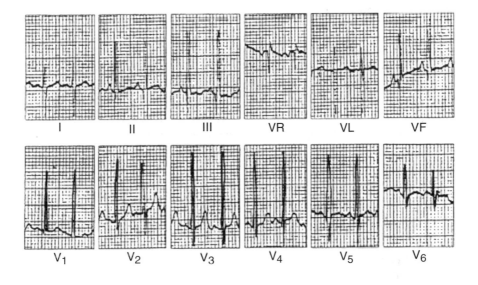

Case 10

This is a non-cyanotic newborn with a systolic 5/6 murmur in the second left intercostal space. Which is the correct diagnosis?

A Ventricular septal defect
B Significant pulmonary stenosis
C Atrial septal defect
D Mitral regurgitation

Answer to Case 10

Comment. The correct diagnosis is a significant pulmonary stenosis in a newborn. Note the qR morphology with a positive T wave in V1 and an RS complex with a positive T wave in V6, typical of a significant RVE in the newborn (p. 40). The ECG corresponds to a pure RVE, as seen in the cases with a severe pulmonary stenosis. A ventricular septal defect generates an ECG with a biventricular enlargement, while mitral regurgitation gives rise to a left ventricular enlargement (LVE). On the other hand, an atrial septal defect generates an rSR' morphology in V1, but never, especially at this age, is there a pure R wave with a positive T wave in V1. Therefore, the correct answer is B (see p. 41).

B

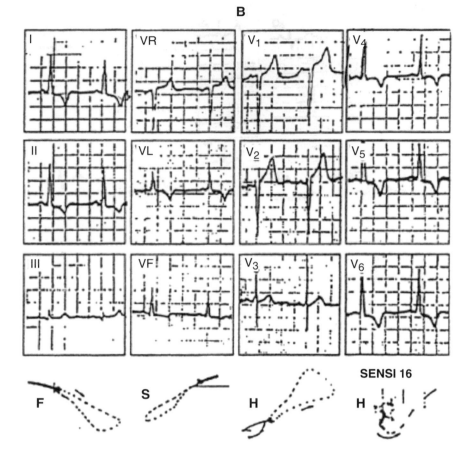

Case 11

This is a 55-year-old patient with a known heart disease evolving during more than 30 years. Which is the correct diagnosis? (ECG is shown at half voltage.)

A Wolff–Parkinson–White syndrome

B Complete left bundle branch block

C Significant left ventricular enlargement

D Mild left ventricular enlargement

Answer to Case 11

Comment. This is the ECG of a patient with a severe and long-standing aortic valve disease (the ECG is shown at half voltage). The QRS complex morphology in lead V6 is a pure R wave (36 mm) with a pattern of strain (ST-segment depression and negative T wave). A myocardial biopsy performed during the valve replacement procedure showed a significant degree of septal fibrosis (the first vector is absent). In the VCG (enlarged HP) it is clearly observed how the beginning of ventricular depolarisation is directed anteriorly but to the left, which explains the absence of a q wave in V5 and V6. Thus, this is the case of significant and long-standing left ventricular enlargement. No criteria for left atrial enlargement are met in this recording; the P wave is rather small probably due to the presence of atrial fibrosis, even though the left atrium is enlarged. The other possibilities are easily ruled out. The PR interval is normal (therefore, it is not a Wolff–Parkinson–White syndrome), the QRS complex duration is less than 120 ms (therefore, it is not a complete left bundle branch block) and the ST–T morphology is typical of a significant, and not mild, left ventricular enlargement. In fact, the ST–T morphology corresponds to a strain pattern with a mixed component (a quite negative and rather symmetric T wave in V4). This patient does not suffer from coronary artery disease and, in the absence of ischaemic heart disease, this repolarisation abnormality supports the severity of the valve heart disease. Therefore, the correct answer is C (see p. 44 and Figure 37).

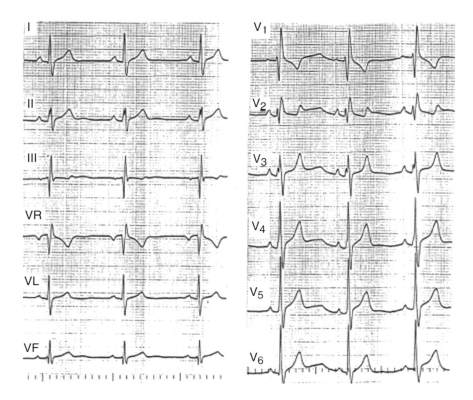

Case 12

This is a 30-year-old patient with an rsR′ morphology in V1. Which is the correct diagnosis?

A Right ventricular enlargement + partial right bundle branch block of the type seen in the atrial septal defect

B Right bundle branch block of new onset due to a pulmonary embolism

C Isolated complete right bundle branch block

D Brugada's syndrome

Answer to Case 12

Comment. This is a 30-year-old patient with a systolic murmur, which was diagnosed during childhood, of atrial septal defect, with a typical morphology of partial right bundle branch block in V1 (QRS < 0.12 seconds). Thus, even the morphology is of the rSR' type in V1, it does not constitute a complete right bundle branch block. The R' wave higher than 10 mm in the presence of a partial right bundle branch block morphology suggests the diagnosis of an associated right ventricular enlargement. On the other hand, the ÂP is close to +30° and the P wave is peaked, mainly in the precordial leads, frequently observed in the cases of right atrial enlargement due to congenital diseases. In the cases with pulmonary embolism, the bundle branch block, if present, is usually of a complete degree and is accompanied by sinus tachycardia and negative T waves from V1 to V3. This QRS morphology is not seen in lead V1 in Brugada's syndrome (there is usually ST-segment elevation with or without R' wave). Therefore, the correct answer is A (see p. 55 and Figure 32B).

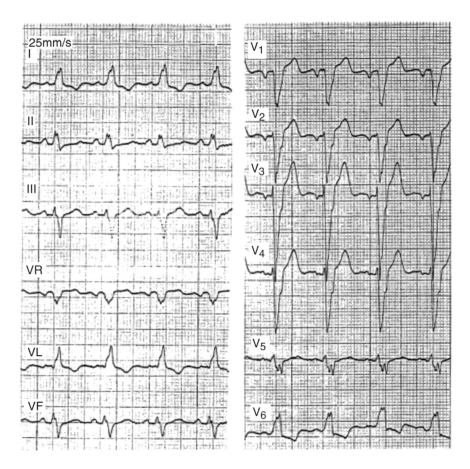

Case 13

This is a 45-year-old patient with signs of heart failure and poor ventricular function. Which is the correct diagnosis?

A Partial left bundle branch block

B Complete left bundle branch block in a patient with a dilated cardiomyopathy, probably of the ischaemic type

C Isolated complete left bundle branch block

D Type-I Wolff–Parkinson–White syndrome

Answer to Case 13

Comment. This is a 45-year-old patient who was diagnosed with dilated cardiomyopathy (Ejection Fraction = 30%). The complete left bundle branch block is atypical, showing a wide QRS complex with slurrings in almost the entire complex (mainly in the ascending QRS slope) and an ÂQRS shifted to the left (−20°). The PR interval is normal, which rules out the diagnosis of a Wolff–Parkinson–White syndrome, and the QRS complex is not positive until V6, which has been suggested as being an indirect sign of right ventricle dilation, just as in this case. Furthermore, there is evidence in this case of biatrial enlargement in the P wave (ÂP shifted to the right, wide bimodal and negative P wave in V1), which supports a diagnosis of dilated cardiomyopathy. A complete left bundle branch block can mask a necrosis Q wave in patients with myocardial infarction. In patients with coronary artery disease and left bundle branch block, the presence of evident notches in the ascending S wave slope supports the diagnosis of a dilated cardiomyopathy secondary to ischaemic heart disease. Therefore, the correct answer is B (see p. 58).

Case 14

This is a 34-year-old patient with frequent paroxysmal arrhythmia crises. Which is the correct diagnosis?

A Lateral myocardial infarction

B Type-III Wolff–Parkinson–White syndrome

C Right ventricular enlargement

D Complete right bundle branch block

Answer to Case 14

Comment. This is a type-III Wolff–Parkinson–White syndrome (short PR interval + delta wave) that mimics an inferolateral infarction (Q wave in leads III and VF and tall R wave in V1–V2). The PR segment is short and the delta wave is directed, mainly, anteriorly. Therefore, there is no possibility of the other diagnoses. The correct answer is B (see p. 63 and Figure 50).

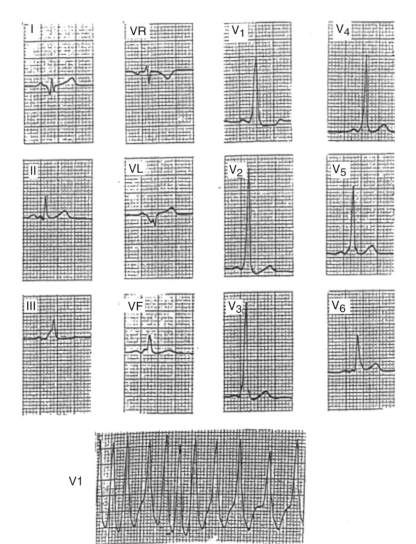

Case 15

This is a 46-year-old patient with frequent paroxysmal arrhythmia crises (see the recording at the bottom). Which is the correct diagnosis?

A Lateral myocardial infarction + ventricular tachycardia

B Type-IV Wolff–Parkinson–White syndrome + paroxysmal atrial fibrillation

C Right ventricular enlargement

D Right bundle branch block + right ventricular enlargement

Answer to Case 15

Comment. This is a patient with a type-IV Wolff–Parkinson–White syndrome (short PR segment + delta wave) that mimics a lateral infarction. The short PR segment and the delta wave are clearly seen. The pre-excitation is directed from left to right (q wave in leads I and VL and tall R wave in V1) (type IV). Additionally, this patient suffers from paroxysmal atrial fibrillation with preexcited complexes that may mimic ventricular tachycardia (bottom). Therefore, the correct answer is B (see Figures 50 and 53).

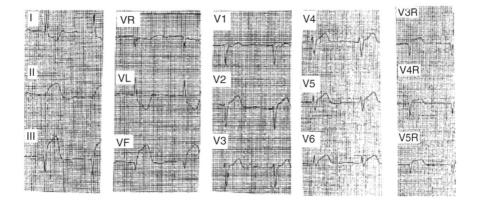

Case 16

This is a patient who suffered a myocardial infarction 2 days ago, and received early therapy with fibrinolytic agents. The ST-segment elevation in the acute phase was located in leads II, III and VF, with a more significant ST elevation in lead III than in II; ST-segment depression is found in lead I and ST-segment elevation is observed in the extreme right precordial leads. Which is the artery involved in this infarction?

A Distal right coronary artery

B Dominant right coronary artery proximal to the right ventricle branch

C Proximal left circumflex coronary artery

D Distal left circumflex coronary artery

Answer to Case 16

Comment. This is a typical ACS involving the inferior wall in the hyperacute phase with low lateral extension (ST-segment elevation in V6). This ECG is not secondary to the occlusion of the left circumflex (Cx) coronary artery, but a dominant right coronary artery (RCA) proximal to the right ventricle branch. This is based on the following reasons: the injury vector, in this case, is directed to the right and is seen as negative in lead I (ST-segment depression). ST-segment elevation is observed in leads III > II, with a mirror image in leads I and VL (>6 mm) (ST-segment depression (VL > I)) and ST elevation in V6. The absence of ST-segment depression is seen in V1 with ST elevation in V2 and in the extreme right precordial leads. Therefore, the correct answer is B (see Figure 74).

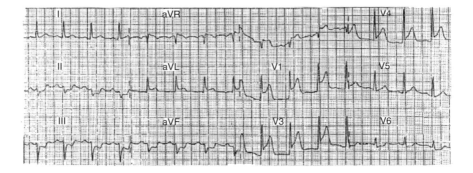

Case 17

This is a 55-year-old patient with an acute coronary syndrome involving the anteroseptal wall (ST-segment elevation in leads V1 through V5 and in VR and VL) and an evident ST-segment depression that is apparent in leads II, III, VF and V6. Give your comments, and your opinion, regarding the characteristics of the occluded artery and the localisation of the stenotic lesion.

A Proximal occlusion of the left anterior descending coronary artery before the take-off of the first diagonal and first septal branches

B Occlusion of the left anterior descending coronary artery proximal to the take-off of the first diagonal branch, but distal to the take-off of the first septal branch

C Occlusion of the left anterior descending coronary artery distal to the take-off of the first diagonal branch and the first septal branch

D Occlusion of the first diagonal branch

Answer to Case 17

Comment. In a patient with an acute coronary syndrome involving the anteroseptal wall (ST-segment elevation in V1–V4), the presence of an ST-segment depression in leads II, III and VF is observed in the cases of occlusion proximal to the take-off of the first diagonal branch (D_1). This occurs as a consequence of the large myocardial mass involved that generates an injury vector that is directed anteriorly and upwards and, therefore, generates an ST-segment elevation in leads V1–V2 to V4–V5 and an ST-segment depression in leads II, III and VF (see Figure 58). The fact that an ST-segment elevation exists in VR and V1, quite evident in this case (> 2 mm), also suggests that the occlusion is located proximal to the first septal branch (S_1). In this case, as in the present situation, an ST-segment depression is also recorded in lead V6 as a mirror image of the elevation in leads VR and V1. Even though the left anterior descending coronary artery is long and wraps the apex, an injury in the inferior area never counterbalances the superior direction of the vector in the cases with a proximal occlusion of the left descending anterior (LAD) coronary artery. Therefore, an ST-segment depression is always found in leads II, III and VF in the case of proximal LAD occlusion. Due to the occurrence of an ST-segment elevation in V1 (> 2.5 mm), it can be assured that the occlusion is located not only proximal to the take-off of D_1, but also proximal to the take-off of the first septal branch (S_1). Therefore, the correct answer is A (see Figures 58 and 73).

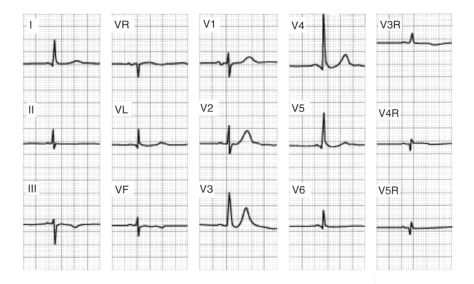

Case 18

This is a 62-year-old patient with an acute myocardial infarction that occurred
1 month ago. Which is the infarction location?

A Impossible to locate
B Isolated inferior
C Isolated lateral
D Inferolateral

Answer to Case 18

Comment. This is a typical lateral infarction. An RS morphology >0.5 is observed in lead V1 with a symmetric positive T wave, with no Q wave in the inferior leads, but with an apparent Q wave in the leads of the back (V7–V9). In this case the correlation with the imaging techniques, especially the nuclear magnetic resonance imaging (MRI) with gadolinium enhancement, shows that there is generally a lateral wall involvement, mainly segments 5 and 11. Generally, the occluded artery is the oblique marginal coronary artery or for short LCX. Due to the heart walls' location within the thorax, in the cases of lateral involvement the vector of necrosis faces V1 and may be seen as RS morphology in this lead. The leads located on the back aid in the diagnosis (qr morphology). Therefore, the correct answer is C (see Figure 59 and Table 16).

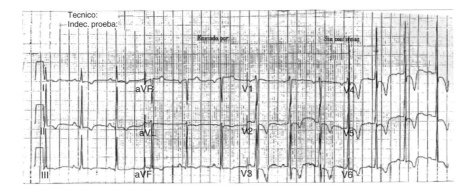

Case 19

This is an asymptomatic 35-year-old patient, with no abnormal findings on physical examination. In your opinion, which is the diagnosis?

A Severe aortic stenosis
B Hypertrophic cardiomyopathy
C Athlete
D Ischaemic heart disease

Answer to Case 19

Comment. The ECG shows large QRS voltage in the left-sided leads with a tall R wave, so the diagnosis of LVE is evident. However, this is not the typical ECG recording of a patient with a severe aortic stenosis (there is a clear negative T wave starting in V2 onwards) nor a patient with ischaemic heart disease (too many negative asymmetric T waves in an asymptomatic patient). The recording is suggestive of a hypertrophic cardiomyopathy with apical predominance, even though ECGs with these characteristics have been recorded in athletes with no hypertrophic cardiomyopathy. This patient is not an athlete, and the echocardiography shows the presence (septum of 18 mm) of a non-obstructive hypertrophic cardiomyopathy. Therefore, the correct answer is B (see p. 117).

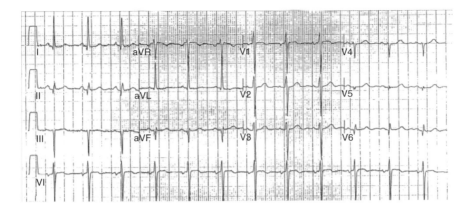

Case 20

This is a 65-year-old patient complaining of palpitations. No chest pain is re-
ferred. Which is the correct diagnosis?

A Normal variant
B Chronic lateral infarction
C Hypertrophic cardiomyopathy
D Heart displaced by a large left pleural effusion

Answer to Case 20

Comment. This ECG is clearly pathologic. No normal variant can explain the morphology seen in V4–V6 with the absence of R wave in V5 and the appearance of a low-voltage QS or QR pattern in V6 and Q wave in inferior leads. Additionally, it is not suggestive of a chronic inferior and/or lateral necrosis because the repolarisation in inferior and V4–V6 is normal and, also, the Q wave is not wide. Rather, this recording might be explained by the presence of an anomalous septal vector that is a consequence of hypertrophied septum and that is directed upwards, to the left and, somewhat, anteriorly (it is positive in leads I, VL, V1, and negative in II, III, V5–V6). The echocardiographic study confirms the diagnosis of non-obstructive hypertrophic cardiomyopathy (septal thickness of 21 mm). Therefore, the correct answer is C (see p. 117 and Table 17).

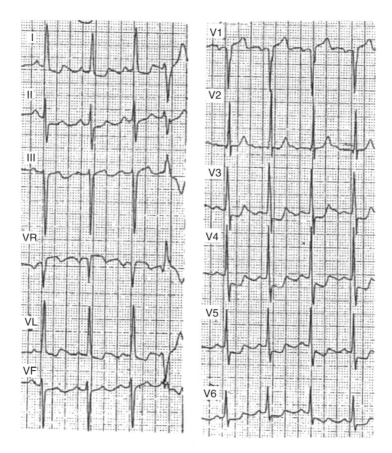

Case 21

This is an ECG of a 67-year-old male patient who has presented several rest angina crises during the last hours, lasting over 30 minutes (acute coronary syndrome). He was then admitted in the Coronary Care Unit. This ECG recording is frequently seen in acute coronary syndromes presenting with involvement of one of the following coronary arteries:

A Proximal right coronary artery

B Left main or equivalent (proximal left anterior descending coronary artery plus proximal circumflex coronary artery)

C Two-vessel disease (right coronary artery plus left anterior descending coronary artery)

D Proximal left anterior descending coronary artery

Answer to Case 21

Comment. This ECG suggests the involvement of the left main trunk or equivalent due to the following facts: (1) ST-segment depression in many leads with and without dominant R wave (I, II, VL, VF and from V3 to V6 with the maximum depression in V3 and V4); (2) ST-segment elevation in VR and V1. Also, a qR morphology is seen in premature ventricular complexes in some leads, as well as a slight ST-segment elevation in the presence of a dominant R wave, which is never observed in normal individuals (see VR). The coronary angiogram showed the involvement of the left main, with a 70% occlusion, of the proximal left anterior descending coronary artery (90%), and of the proximal circumflex coronary artery (80%). Surgical revascularisation was urgently carried out. Therefore, the correct answer is B (see Figure 76 and p. 92).

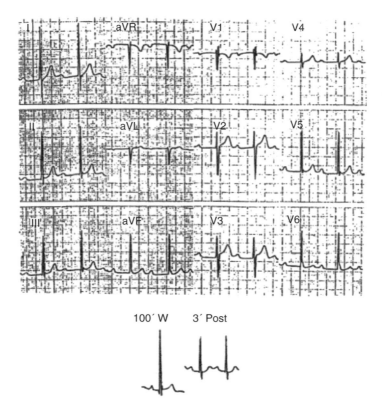

100´ W   3´ Post

Case 22

This is from a 34-year-old patient, athlete, asymptomatic, presenting during a check-up with tall QRS complexes in V5–V6 with a positive T wave, rSr' in V1 and the first-degree atrioventricular block in the ECG. Which is the correct diagnosis?

A Normal variant in an athlete; the nocturnal and during exercise response of the first-degree atrioventricular block should be assessed

B The V1 morphology advises to rule out Brugada's pattern

C Biventricular enlargement

D Right bundle branch block, supported by the presence of a rsr' morphology in V1

Answer to Case 22

Comment. Physical examination is normal. It is evident that the patient presents features that are quite typical of an athlete's ECG. The PR interval is long and V1 shows rsr' morphology with a narrow r' wave and no ST-segment elevation, which rules out the diagnosis of Brugada's pattern. Biventricular enlargement seems unlikely, since although a high QRS complex voltage is present, repolarisation is not very abnormal. The QRS is narrow and the rsr' in V1 is found often in athletes without evident right ventricle (RV) hypertrophy or RBBB, but with some delay of activation of basal part of the RV. On the whole, the ECG could be normal for an athlete. The performance of an exercise stress test to evaluate the PR interval behaviour seems the most correct action. Given the test was done, and the PR interval normalised, though at 3 minutes following exercise, it began to lengthen again. Naturally, a Holter study to check for severe bradyarrhythmias and an echocardiogram could well be indicated. A marked nocturnal sinus bradycardia with an even larger PR interval was the only finding in the Holter study in this case. The echocardiogram shows normal right and left ventricles. Therefore, the correct answer is A (see p. 117).

References

1 Bayés de Luna A. Clinical Electrocardiography: A Textbook. 2nd edition. New York: Futura, 1999.

2 Moss A. A renaissance in electrocardiography. Ann Noninvasive Electrocardiol 2004; 9: 1–2.

3 Cranefield PF. The Conduction of the Cardiac Impulse. Mount Kisco, NY: Future Publ. Co., 1975.

4 Grant RP. Clinical Electrocardiography: The Spatial Vector Approach. New York: McGraw-Hill, 1957.

5 McFarlane P, Veitch Lawrie TD (eds). Comprehensive Electrocardiography. Oxford: Pergamon Press, 1989.

6 Cabrera E. Teoría y Práctica de la Electrocardiografía. Mexico, DF: La Prensa Médica Mexicana, 1958.

7 Sodi D, Bisteni A, Medrano G. Electrocardiografía y Vectorcardiografía Deductivas. Vol. 1. Mexico, DF: La Prensa Médica Mexicana, 1964.

8 Durrer D, Van Dam R, Freud G, Janse M, Meijler F, Arzbaecher R. Total excitation of the isolated human heart. Circulation 1970; 41: 899–912.

9 Savelieva I, Yi G, Guo X, Hnatkova K, Malik M. Agreement and reproducibility of automatic versus manual measurement of QT interval and QT dispersion. Am J Cardiol 1998; 81: 471–477.

10 Moss AJ. Long QT syndrome. JAMA 2003; 289: 2041–2044.

11 Yap YG, Camm AJ. Drug induced QT prolongation and torsades de pointes. Heart 2003; 89: 1363–1372.

12 Gaita F, Giustetto C, Bianchi F, Wolpert C, Schimpf R, Riccardi R, et al. Short QT syndrome: a familial cause of sudden death. Circulation 2003; 108: 965–970.

13 Puech P. L'activite Électrique Auriculaire Normale e Pathologique. Paris: Masson, 1956.

14 Zimmermann HA. The Auricular Electrocardiogram. Springfield: Charles C. Thomas Publ., 1968.

15 Josephson ME, Kastor JA, Morganroth J. ECG left atrial enlargement. Electrophysiologic, echocardiographic and hemodynamic correlations. Am J Cardiol 1977; 39: 967–971.

16 Bayés de Luna A, Fort de Ribot R, Trilla E, Julia J, García J, Sadurni J, et al. Electrocardiographic and vectorcardiographic study of interatrial conduction disturbances with left atrial retrograde activation. J Electrocardiol 1985; 18: 1–13.

17 Bayés de Luna A, Cladellas M, Oter R, Guindo J, Torres P, Marti V, et al. Interatrial conduction block and retrograde activation of the left atrium and paroxysmal supraventricular tachyarrhythmias. Eur Heart J 1988; 9: 1112–1118.

18 Bayés de Luna A, Guindo J, Viñolas X, Martinez Rubio A, Oter R, Bayes Genis A. Third degree inter-atrial block and supraventricular tachyarrhythmias. Europace 1999; 1: 3–6.

19 Bayés de Luna A, Serra Genís C, Guix M, Trilla E. Septal fibrosis as determinant of Q waves in patients with aortic valve disease. Eur Heart J 1983; 4(Suppl. E): 86.

20 Cabrera E, Monroy JR. Systolic and diastolic loading of the heart. ECG data. Am Heart J 1952; 43: 669–686.

21 Wagner G. Marriot's Practical Electrocardiography. 10th edition. New York: Lippincott Williams and Wilkins, 2001.

22 Horan LG, Flowers NC. ECG and VCG. In Braunwald E (ed) Heart Disease. Philadelphia, PA: WB Saunders, 1980.

23 Lenegre J, Moreau PH. Le bloc auriculo-ventriculaire chronique. Etude anatomique, clinique et histologique. Arch Mal Coeur 1963; 56: 867–888.

24 Rosenbaum MB, Elizari MV, Lazzari JO. Los Hemibloqueos. Buenos Aires: Ed. Paidos, 1968.

25 Bayés de Luna A, Torner P, Oter R, Oca F, Guindo J, Rivera I, et al. Study of the evolution of masked bifascicular block. PACE 1989; 11: 1517.

26 Wolff L, Parkinson J, White DD. Bundle branch block with short PR interval in healthy young people prone to paroxysmal tachycardia. Am Heart J 1930; 5: 685.

27 Lown B, Ganong WF, Levine SA. The syndrome of short PR interval, normal QRS complex and paroxysmal rapid heart beat. Circulation 1957; 5: 693–706.

28 Wellens HJJ, Attie J, Smeets J, Cruz F, Gorgels A, Brugada P. The ECG in patients with multiple accessory pathways. JACC 1990; 16: 745–751.

29 Milstein S, Sharma AD, Guiraudon GM, Klein GJ. An algorithm for the electrocardiographic localization of accessory pathways is the Wolff–Parkinson–White syndrome. PACE 1987; 10: 555–563.

30 Montoya PT, Brugada P, Smeets J, Talajic M, Della Bella P, Lezaun R, et al. Ventricular fibrillation in the Wolff–Parkinson–White syndrome. Eur Heart J 1991; 12: 144–150.

31 Bayés de Luna A, Carreras F, Cygankiewicz I, Leta R, Flotats A, Carrió I, et al. Evolving myocardial infarction with ST elevation: anatomic consideration regarding the correlation between the site of occlusion and injured segments of the heart. Ann Noninvasive Electrocardiol 2004; 9: 71–77.

32 Cerqueira MD, Weissman NJ, Disizian V, Jacobs AK, Kaul S, Laskey WK, et al. Standardized myocardial segmentation and nomenclature for tomographic imaging of the heart. A statement for healthcare professionals from the Cardiac Imaging Committee of the Council on Clinical Cardiology of the American Heart Association. Circulation 2002; 105: 539–542.

33 Bayés de Luna A, Wagner G, Birnbaum Y, Nikus K, Fiol M, Gorgels A, et al. A new terminology for the left ventricular walls and for the locations of Q wave and Q wave equivalent myocardial infarcts based on the standard of cardiac magnetic resonance imaging. Circulation 2006; 114:1755–1760.

34 Bayés de Luna A, Cino JM, Pujadas S, Cygankiewicz I, Carreras F, Garcia-Moll X, et al. Concordance of electrocardiographic patterns and healed myocardial infarction location detected by cardiovascular magnetic resonance. Am J Cardiol 2006; 97: 443–451.

35 Cino JM, Pujadas S, Carreras F, Cygankiewicz I, Leta R, Noguero M, et al. Utility of contrast-enhanced cardiovascular magnetic resonance (CE-CMR) to assess how likely is an infarct to produce a typical ECG pattern. Journal of Cardiovascular Magnetic Resonance 2006; 8: 335–344.

36 Hathaway WR, Peterson ED, Wagner GS, Granger CB, Zabel KH, Pieper KS, et al. Prognostic significance of the initial electrocardiogram in patients with acute myocardial infarction. GUSTO-I Investigators. Global Utilization of Streptokinase and t-PA for Occluded Coronary Arteries. JAMA 1998; 279: 38–91.

37 Wellens HJ, Gorgels A, Doevendans PA. The ECG in Acute Myocardial Infarction and Unstable Angina. Boston: Kluwer, 2003.

38 Sclarowsky S. Electrocardiography of Acute Myocardial Ischemia. London: Martin Dunitz, 1999.

39 Bayés de Luna A, Antman E, Fiol M. The Role of 12-Lead ECG in ST Elevation MI. Oxford: Blackwell Publishing 2006.

40 Fiol M, Cygankiewicz I, Bayés Genis A, Carrillo A, Santoya O, Gómez A, *et al.* The value of ECG algorithm based on 'ups and downs' of ST in assessment of a culprit artery in evolving inferior myocardial infarction. Am J Cardiol 2004; 94: 709–714.

41 Fiol M, Carrillo A, Cygankiewicz I, Ayestaran J, Caldes O, Peral V, *et al.* New criteria based on ST changes in 12 leads surface ECG to detect proximal vs distal right coronary artery occlusion in case of an acute inferoposterior myocardial infarction. Ann Noninvasive Electrocardiol 2004; 9(4): 383–388.

42 Sadanandan S, Hochman S, Kolodziej A, Criger D, Ros A, Selvester R, *et al.* Clinical and angiographic characteristics of patients with combined anterior and inferior ST segment elevation in the initial ECG during acute myocardial infarction. Am Heart J 2003; 146: 653–661.

43 Yamaji H, Iwasaki K, Kusachi S, Murakami T, Hirami R, Hamamoto H, *et al.* Prediction of acute left main coronary artery obstruction by 12-lead electrocardiography. ST segment elevation in lead VR with less ST segment elevation in lead V1. J Am Coll Cardiol 2001; 48: 1348–1354.

44 Nikus KC, Escola MJ, Virtanen VK, Vikman S, Niemela KO, Huhtala H, *et al.* ST depression with negative T waves in leads V4–V5 – a marker of a severe coronary artery disease in non-ST elevation acute coronary syndrome: a prospective study of angina at rest with troponin, clinical, electrocardiographic, and angiographic correlation. Ann Noninvasive Electrocardiol 2004; 9: 207–214.

45 Bayés de Luna A, Carreras F, Cladellas M, Oca F, Sagues F, Garcia Moll M. Holter ECG study of the electrocardiographic phenomena in Prinzmetal angina attacks with emphasis on the study of ventricular arrhythmias. J Electrocardiol 1985; 18: 267–275.

46 Goldberger M. Myocardial Infarction: ECG Differential diagnosis. St Louis, MO: Mosby Co., 1975.

47 Phibbs B, Marcus F, Marriott HJ, Moss A, Spodick DH. Q-wave versus non-Q wave myocardial infarction: a meaningless distinction. J Am Coll Cardiol 1999; 33: 576–582.

48 Schamroth L. The electrocardiology of coronary artery disease. Oxford: Blackwell Scientific Publications, 1975.

49 Myocardial infarction redefined – a consensus document of The Joint European Society of Cardiology/American College of Cardiology Committee for the redefinition of myocardial infarction. Eur Heart J 2000; 21: 1502–1513.

50 Wagner GS, Bahit MC, Criger D, Bayés de Luna A, Chaitman B, Clemmensen P, *et al.* Toward a new definition of acute myocardial infarction for the 21st century: Status of the ESC/ACC consensus conference. J Electrocardiol 2000; 33(Suppl.): 57–9.

51 Bogaty P, Boyer L, Rousseau L, Arsenault M. Is anteroseptal myocardial infarction an appropriate term? Am J Med 2002; 113: 37–41.

52 Selvanayagam JB, Kardos A, Nicolson D, Francis J, Petersen SE, Robson M, *et al.* Anteroseptal and apical myocardial infarction: a controversy addressed using delayed enhancement cardiovascular magnetic resonance imaging. J Cardiovasc Magn Res 2004; 6: 653–661.

53 Moon JCC, Perez de Arenaza P, Elkington AG, Taneja AK, John AS, Wang D, *et al.* The pathologic basis of Q wave and non-Q wave myocardial infarction. A cardiovascular magnetic resonance study. J Am Coll Cardiol 2004; 44: 554–560.

54 Das MK, Khan B, Jacob S, Kumar A, Mahenthiran J. Significance of a fragmented QRS complex versus a Q wave in patients with coronary artery disease. Circulation 2006; 113(21): 2495–2501.

55 Selvester RH, Wagner GS, Hindman NB. The Selvester QRS scoring system for estimating myocardial infarction size: the development and application of the system. Arch Int Med 1985; 145: 1877–1881.

56 Engblom H, Wagner GS, Sester RM, Selvester RH, Billgren T, Kasper JM, *et al.* Quantitative clinical assessment of chronic anterior myocardial infarction with delayed enhancement magnetic resonance imaging and QRS scoring. Am Heart J 2003; 146: 359–366.

57 Bayés de Luna A, Fiol-Sala M. The ECG of ischemic heart disease: clinical and imaging correlations and prognostic implications. London: Blackwell, 2007.

58 Sgarbossa EB, Pinski SL, Barbagelata A, Underwood DA, Gates KB, Topol EJ, *et al.* Electrocardiographic diagnosis of evolving acute myocardial infarction in the presence of left bundle-branch block. GUSTO-1 (Global Utilization of Streptokinase and Tissue Plasminogen Activator for Occluded Coronary Arteries) Investigators. N Engl J Med 1996; 334: 481.

59 Wackers F, Lie KL, David G, Durrer D, Wellens HJJ. Assessment of the value of the ECG signs for myocardial infarction in left bundle branch block by Thallium. Am J Cardiol 1978; 41: 428.

60 Sgarbossa E, Pinski S, Gates K, Wagner G. Early ECG diagnosis of acute myocardial infarction in the presence of ventricular paced rhythm. Am J Cardiol 1996; 77: 423–424.

61 Antzelevitch Ch, Brugada P, Brugada J, Brugada R. The Brugada Syndrome. London: Blackwell-Futura, 2005.

62 Cosin J, Gimeno JV, Ramirez A, Bayés de Luna A, Martín G, Blas E. Aproximación experimental al estudio de los bloqueos parietales del ventrículo derecho. Rev Esp Card 1983; 36: 125–132.

63 Birnbaum Y, Atar S. Electrocardiogram risk stratification of non-ST elevation acute coronary syndrome. J Electrocardiology 2006; 39: 558–560.

64 Surawicz B. Relationship between electrocardiogram and electrolytes. Am Heart J 1967; 73: 814–834.

Index